'Bill Ford offers valuable advice as to how to make life easier, fuller, and certainly more enjoyable. A worthwhile book'
Susan Jeffers, Ph.D, bestselling author of *Feel the Fear and do it Anyway* and *Embracing Uncertainty*

'With humour, warmth and dash of self-deprecation, Bill Ford whips up a feast for those craving more energy and the feeling of being fully alive. With practical stories and tips this book will really show you how to fill up your life's energy tank and keep it full without making yourself busier in the process'
Laura Berman Fortgang, author of *Living Your Best Life* and *Take Yourself to the Top*

'This book will make a world of difference for anyone who finds they are running the treadmill and not achieving break-through results in their lives. I looked forward to a few quiet moments to complete the exercises in the back. This should be required reading for anyone on the go and wanting more'
Cynder Niemela, Executive and Team Coach, co-author *Leading High Impact Teams: The Coach Approach to Peak Performance*

'This book is changing the way I live and work'
Nancy Kline, President, Time To Think Inc.

HIGH ENERGY HABITS

The Busy Person's Guide
To More Energy
(without diets or exercise)

BILL FORD

POCKET
BOOKS

LONDON · SYDNEY · NEW YORK · TOKYO · SINGAPORE · TORONTO

First published in Great Britain by Pocket Books, 2002
An imprint of Simon & Schuster UK Ltd
A Viacom Company

3 5 7 9 10 8 6 4 2

Simon & Schuster UK Ltd
Africa House
64–78 Kingsway
London WC2B 6AH

www.simonsays.co.uk

Simon & Schuster Australia
Sydney

A CIP catalogue record for this book is available from the British Library

ISBN 0-7434-2894-3

Typeset by Palimpsest Book Production Limited,
Polmont, Stirlingshire
Printed and bound in Great Britain by
Bookmarque Ltd, Croydon

*Unless otherwise indicated, clients' names have
been changed to maintain confidentiality.*

ACKNOWLEDGEMENTS

My heartfelt thanks to the following for supporting me in bringing this book to life:

Nancy Kline for startling me by pointing out that my workshop was a book.

Thomas Leonard, Sandy Vilas and Coach U for their generosity and wealth of ideas and without whom a large part of this book would not have existed.

Amanda Seyderhelm, my agent and writing coach, for helping me make this a reality quickly.

For helping me in a variety of ways to make the book, and in the process of producing it, better than it might otherwise have been: Mark Wilson, John Pickston, Andrea Millwood-Hargrave, Denise Turner, Jane Marquis, Laura Berman Fortgang, Nigel Marsh, the staff at The New Learning Centre, Aboodi Shaby, Mike Turner, Paul Berman, Bridget Postlethwaite, Talane Miedaner, Philip Lamba, Joanna Ludlum, Anup Chib, Nick Reed, Alice Liftin, Mike Neill, Roger and Sally Jarman, the participants at my workshops, my clients and colleagues.

Lastly, my wife Rosemary for your encouragement, sound judgement, enthusiasm, patience and unfailing support.

CONTENTS

FOREWORD

This book is changing the way I live and work. What Bill says about increasing energy is true. And of the thirty or so specific ways he suggests we do things differently, in order to increase energy and to stop energy drain, nineteen of them applied to me, bull's-eye. Others I was already doing to some degree, but did not realise that doing them increases energy.

That is the key contribution of this book. Bill has observed what we are all doing and not doing; he has understood those things in the context of energy; and he has, therefore, transformed our relationship to those things. It is the energy concept that is so exciting.

To be specific: I have increasingly over the past year found that even though I have developed my life's work, am following the passion and vision I know is from my core, taking the right level of risk and being happy, I have begun to feel inexplicably tired lots of the time. I also have begun to wonder why I do not seem to be able consistently to do each day what I know needs to be done on the big projects until time deadlines kick off their particular adrenaline-powered, exhausting brand of focus and resolve. This has made me curious at best and, if I am honest, a bit worried.

Then I read this book. It helped me see that energy would come from changing my relationship to the little things and from making small changes that would have a huge effect. I could see, for example, that energy would come from doing things I had been putting off, both the nagging things I dreaded and those I felt guilty for doing because they gave me pleasure. I could see that fixing problems by giving them more time and that consistently allowing enough time to be early to appointments were not just wise practices by the very together people I tried to emulate, but would also actually increase my energy. I began also to see that contact with people need not be lengthy to be meaningful *and* energising. I already knew that slowing down speeds things up, but now I could see that doing it would also generate energy for me.

This energy connection, this understanding about what increases energy, has lifted many of the formerly bewildering pieces of my life into a new realm of comprehension and joy. And in a sense, understanding the energy context has given me permission to do things guilt-free, with pleasure and vitality.

Bill's insights have also shone a light on my own work, The Thinking Environment™. I see now that not only do the Ten Components of a Thinking Environment™ make it possible for people to think for themselves brilliantly, they also enormously increase the physical energy of people as they apply them. Wonderful. I shall teach this dimension from now on.

It is a great relief, a liberation really, to relate to the myriad activities, relationships and engagements in my life from this fresh and true perspective of energy gain.

Bill's ideas are readily absorbed both because of the integrity and workability of them, and also because of the warmth and acceptance of each of us that comes through in his writing. His style is consistent with his theory: to be appreciated, accepted and encouraged, rather than blamed, criticised or pressured, increases self esteem which leads to more energy.

What a welcome addition his ideas are in our relentlessly busy lives. I admire, in particular, Bill's ability to see what is right in front of us, understand it, and hand it gently back to us so that we can see it, too.

Nancy Kline
President, Time To Think™, Inc.

INTRODUCTION

Would you like to have more energy? Would you like to wake up in the morning looking forward to what the day will bring, and to reach the evening with energy in reserve? Would you like to feel calmer, more in control, more able to enjoy life? It's easier to achieve than you think:

> Do less of what drains your energy and more of what boosts your energy.

Can it be that simple? Well, yes it can. Start by noticing which things reduce your energy and which increase it. Then take some small steps to reduce those that drain your energy and to boost those that enhance it.

I can imagine that some of you will have lots of objections and sound reasons as to why this may not work for you, but humour me. I will explain the practical steps necessary to make the changes, and the effort involved will repay itself many times over. Your life may be just about to change gear.

A lot of the people I meet are successful, yet even so they often experience a feeling of being overwhelmed. They feel that life is tough and, frankly, not that much fun. There seem to be many causes: a 'To Do' list that never gets shorter; too many demands in their different roles (partner, child, grandchild, parent, fundraiser, sibling, neighbour, employee, manager); too many meetings; too many e-mails; too much travel; too much information to absorb and too easily contacted through mobile communications. They feel a lack of control, are perpetually struggling and never getting closer to the light at the end of the tunnel. Fire-fighting and unreasonable demands have almost become the norm.

It doesn't have to be this way. When you have more energy, you feel more resilient and resourceful. Problems become smaller, are dealt with more completely and recur less often. Life seems more manageable and starts to be a more positive experience. People with more energy attract similar people, are more fun to be around and get more done.

The author

For a long time, I used to have very low energy. It started in childhood growing up with a father who was violent and unpredictable. I learnt then how to form a small target by holding my energy back and maintaining a low profile in order to avoid getting hurt. As an adult, I continued this behaviour and was often slow to contribute in groups, but was not aware of what I was doing or why. This behaviour got me fired, which led me to explore through a variety of means what was going on.

As a result of that exploration, my energy is now much higher and I have learned to notice and act more quickly on the things that impact my energy. I have since been promoted several times, increased profits by several million pounds for my employers and been singled out for spontaneous bonuses and other forms of recognition. For the last seven years, I have run my own business, Coaching Directors. I work as an Executive Coach, have a successful practice and been featured in *The Times*. What follows is based on what I have learned.

HIGH ENERGY PEOPLE

People with high energy are not only more attractive, they seem to have an easier, and better, time than the rest of us. They appear to move through life with less bruising, friction and erosion. Here are some of the words and phrases that have been used to describe people with high energy:

- a spark in the eye
- a certain fluidity
- the mood in a roomful of people changes when they walk in
- somehow attractive – you are drawn to them
- you feel better around them
- openness
- passionate
- self-assured
- robust yet vulnerable
- they seem to accept themselves, warts and all

- they have a sense of humour; a mischievous, playful side
- they seem to have more time
- approachable
- living in the present, not distracted or absent
- have a sense of clarity and purpose about them
- optimistic, with a positive attitude
- spontaneous

By contrast, people with low energy appear:

- hesitant, uncertain
- one-paced
- private
- awkward, sort of angular
- distracted
- fragile
- reserved
- slow to commit, indecisive
- worn down
- pessimistic
- their words lack conviction

Which words or phrases best describe the way you are today? Would you prefer people to describe you more often using phrases from the first group?

And what is a man without energy? Nothing – nothing at all. What is the grandest thing in *Paradise Lost*? – the Archfiend's terrible energy! What was the greatest feature in Napoleon's character? His unconquerable energy! Sum all the gifts that man is endowed with, and we give our greatest share of admiration to his energy. And today if I were a heathen, I would rear a statue to Energy and fall down and worship it!

Mark Twain

This book is NOT about

Some of you will be relieved to find that this book is NOT about diet, nutrients, exercise, chakras, power naps or feng shui. All these things have a contribution to make and there are a gazillion books on them.

This book IS about

This book is more about 'head stuff': paying attention to different things, noticing how you respond to the little things and doing something about them because they matter, often more than they appear to. What I want is for you to feel inspired to take a number of small steps in order to achieve a big benefit. The essence of this book is about bite-sized, straightforward, achievable steps that make a huge difference.

How to read this book

You do not have to read this book from start to finish; feel free to dip in anywhere. You can do the exercises as you go through, do them later or never do them at all. Clearly, if you want to get the full benefit, it makes sense to read the whole book and do the exercises, but you are likely to get a lot from it just by dipping in and reading parts of it.

By the time you finish this book
If you follow the steps in this book, then by the time you finish you will:

- Have repaired all those little things that need fixing, that you've been meaning to get around to, but have been ignoring – it takes energy to ignore them.
- Have cleared the clutter in your life – a big energy drain.
- Spend more time with the people who bring out the best in you.
- Be clear what your natural strengths are and you will use them more often.
- Build in a 'margin' in your life for contingencies, so that when things go wrong the impact is less and any anxiety is reduced. This will increase your sense of resourcefulness and energy.
- Have regular time in your schedule for activities that boost your energy. You will see that these are not optional but rather they recharge your batteries and help you cope with all the demands in your life.
- Change your perspective so that instead of seeing what is wrong you will appreciate what is right and abundant in your life and be able to enjoy your life more.
- Connect with people more often and feel the increased energy that comes from having more positive contact with different people.
- Slow down at times and get more done.
- Find being happy is easier.

- Find it easier and less wearing to deal with children.
- Get more help where you need it and progress will be quicker.
- Notice more quickly what things drain your energy and what boosts it, and want to do something about it.

Case study
One of my coaching clients, Mark Wilson, is an independent financial advisor in Surrey, who was running a successful business before he starting coaching with me. Mark, aged forty, started coaching because he was curious, not because there was anything particular he wanted to fix. We worked on a variety of topics and managing energy was often a core theme. After a year of coaching, he had made several changes in his life:

- He played golf once a week.
- He rarely worked evenings any longer.
- He reconnected with his friends.
- He spent more time with his family.
- He no longer felt that he was 'living in a fog' when he was with his family.
- He felt in complete control.
- His wife said to him spontaneously 'it's like having the old you back again'.
- He reduced his working week from 66 hours on average to 42.

Some of you may be wondering whether this was achieved at the expense of his business. It wasn't: his turnover tripled at the same time as he made all these changes. How did he do it? Firstly, he is a remarkable individual who is very open to new ideas and looks for opportunities to grow. Secondly, he implemented the ideas in this book.

ADDITIONAL BENEFITS

Having more energy affects all areas of life. I asked my clients and the audiences at my workshops what benefits they saw from the steps outlined in the book and this is what they reported:

- They are more aware of how things affect them and they have more sense that they can do something about it.
- They feel more in control and less as if they are behind all the time.
- They enjoy what they do more.
- They get more done.
- The quality of their output improves.
- They achieve improved profits.
- They feel better about the world.
- Problems become easier to deal with.
- They do a little on a regular basis.
- They are more willing to take action.
- Things get done with less effort.
- They stop putting up with unsatisfactory situations.
- They feel more in the present.
- They feel less stressed.
- They have more sense of time.

Having more energy can help us to feel more optimistic. Psychologists have demonstrated that optimism is linked to productivity. One study by the psychologists Seligman and Schulman explored the link between optimism and sales among a group of life insurance salespeople. They used a written test to assess optimism and divided the group into two: those above and below the median – the 'optimists' and the 'pessimists'. They then monitored sales for the two groups over two years.

In the first year, the optimists sold 29 per cent more insurance in their first year than the pessimists. In the second year, the gap widened: the optimists sold 130 per cent more insurance than the pessimists. So feeling more optimistic is not just a nice-to-have. It makes a measurable difference to productivity that is significant and long term.

RATE YOUR ENERGY LEVEL

In order to rate your current energy level, read the following statements. Tick those that apply to you, ignore those that don't and compare your total with the table below. Answer quickly, don't think about it – take the first response that comes.

1. Seeing my friends can seem a huge effort sometimes. ☐
2. I'm always rushing. ☐
3. I rarely stop for lunch. ☐
4. I wake up in the morning feeling tired. ☐
5. My 'To Do' list never gets much shorter. ☐

6. I have no time for exercise. ☐

7. I often can't face going in to work/starting the day. ☐

8. I dread the phone ringing in the evening in case someone wants to chat. ☐

9. My evenings are spent recovering for the next day. ☐

10. At the end of the day I am always tired. ☐

11. All my hobbies are on hold. ☐

12. My time is over-committed. ☐

13. I don't initiate conversations with shop staff. ☐

14. I watch over an hour of television daily. ☐

15. I know I'm not eating properly most of the time. ☐

16. Life feels an uphill struggle most of the time. ☐

17. I go to bed late. ☐

18. If I stopped work my savings would last less than a year. ☐

19. I don't ask for help. ☐

20. I am often late, or almost late. ☐

21. I find it impossible to say 'No'. ☐

22. I often think that there must be more to life than this. ☐

23. I don't pay many compliments to others. ☐

24. I often interrupt others and finish their sentences. ☐

25. My personal files and papers need to be organised. ☐

26. Some of my appliances need repair. ☐

27. It's hard to switch off from work. ☐

28. I am often behind with my tax returns. ☐

29. I often think about what I wish I had said at the time. ☐
30. I prefer to avoid difficult conversations. ☐
31. I am behind with phone calls, letters and e-mails. ☐
32. I don't have enough time to myself. ☐
33. There are lots of little jobs around the house that need attention. ☐
34. I always wait till the petrol tank is dangerously close to empty before I fill up. ☐
35. The inside of my car has not been cleaned for over three months. ☐
36. I rarely see my best friend or don't have one. ☐
37. I do a lot of things I don't enjoy. ☐
38. I am often not happy with my life. ☐
39. I like to sort out my problems by myself. ☐
40. I like to avoid all risks ☐

TOTAL _____

What was your score?
- *5 or less* You have already eliminated many energy drains – this book will be a 'tune up'.
- *6 to 15* You have eliminated some energy drains and have lots of potential for improvement.
- *16 or more* You have many avoidable energy drains and have a huge potential to increase available energy.

Chapter 1

PREPARE WELL

Become more self aware and have higher expectations for your quality of life. Make some attitude shifts to achieve faster progress to more energy.

To get the best out of this book you will need to look at changing some of your attitudes and perspectives. You will be able to get by without doing so, but progress will be much faster if you integrate the points outlined in this chapter. People with high energy view things a little differently, and so can you if you learn to:

- Pay attention to the 'little voice'.
- Be selfish (about self-care).
- Be more assertive about what *you* want.
- Shift from 'Make do' to 'Can do' (give yourself permission to want what *you* want).
- Become more sensitive and pay attention to the details.
- Notice what drains your energy and what increases it.

- Take lots of small steps.
- Take daily action (thinking is not enough).

You may want to dip into this book at different points and try out things in a different order to here – that is fine. The pieces stand alone and build on each other. Allow yourself to come back to ideas that intrigue you. Some of them will make an immediate impression, others will spend some time simmering in the background. Implement them when it feels right for you. You may find that some of the ideas won't work for you in the way described. Don't reject them out of hand – see which bits you like and which you're less sure about. Consider how you might modify them to suit your life better and then implement the modified version. Keep an open mind, even if you disagree, and be willing to experiment.

Since this book is intended for busy people, I have kept it short in the hope that you will feel more able to come back to it to deepen the learning and try out more of the ideas. Sometimes seeing the same thing on a different occasion can make a big difference – we change all the time and it makes sense for our reactions to be different. Give yourself space and time to experience these different reactions.

One thing I strongly suggest you do to make the implementation more certain, is to find a buddy, friend, partner or coach who is willing to work on this material with you. Maybe find someone you would like to spend more time with and suggest you set a theme for the month using one of the chapters and set up regular meetings, by phone if necessary, to keep each other focused, supported and accountable.

PAY ATTENTION TO THE 'LITTLE VOICE'

While I was writing this book a friend e-mailed me to ask what was the single most important way of increasing energy. I had to pause and think for several minutes. In many ways I think it is this: pay attention to the 'little voice'. It is your best friend, and too often ignored. If you listen closely and act on what it says, then the rest will almost sort itself out. One of the challenges is that the voice can easily be drowned out by the noise in our lives.

> There are voices which we hear in solitude, but they grow faint and inaudible as we enter into the world.
> *Ralph Waldo Emerson*

One of my clients sometimes gets a thought to call one of his clients. Often it is someone he intended to call over the next week or so, but he deliberately chooses to respond and calls them immediately. What he has found on a number of occasions is that he gets through to them straightaway and they in turn were thinking of calling him. One benefit for him is that he avoids the potential energy drain of playing phone tag. Responding immediately to his 'little voice' is a way to increase efficiency.

Messages are often repeated with increasing intensity. The sequence (with thanks to coach Pam Richarde) is as follows:

1. Life messages – if you are present and listening to the 'little voice', then you get the chance to extract

and implement the lessons. If you don't deal with them, then you can expect the next level of message.

2. Problems – and if you don't deal with them quickly enough, then you can expect the next level.

3. Crisis – this is a big message that is harder to ignore.

The small messages provide clues several times over on how things could be better and give you the chance to make adjustments now before a more impactful message is necessary. I have noticed that when my wife, Rosemary, is stressed she will accidentally set off the car alarm more often and the rear wheel of the car is more likely to bump into the pavement when cornering. I imagine if she stopped to consider the message of these events, it would be along the lines of 'You are doing too much. Slow down, you need a break. Your next message will be a minor prang. Stay tuned.'

Sometimes we seem to keep ourselves busy, in order not to hear the 'little voice', in case we hear something uncomfortable, awkward or inconvenient. This is usually just a delaying tactic. It is far better to slow down and face the risk of hearing the truth sooner. Stop using activity or busy-ness as an anaesthetic.

If you surround yourself with activity and noise, moving from room to room turning on the TV, radio and CD player in each room to fill the silence, then it will be harder to hear. The fact that it is little does not mean it is insignificant. It is small because we are not used to lis-tening and, unlike some cultures, do not trust it enough. This is the voice of your intuition and it needs nurturing, since it gets so much competition.

So, how do you tune in to this voice? Here are some ideas:

- Sit quietly for 20 minutes doing nothing.
- Meditate.
- Write a journal (*see* Chapter 9).
- Drive without the radio on.
- Cook or do another manual activity, without having the radio on
- Allocate thinking time in your schedule (*see* page 79).

Reverie is not a mind vacuum. It is rather the gift of an hour which knows the plenitude of the soul.

Gaston Bachelard

Experiment with those ideas that you have energy for. Try setting aside a little time to consider what changes have occurred. It may be that you feel calmer, more centred, more focused, more energetic, less stressed, etc. See what emerges for you, but be aware that you may need to do this exercise more than once to detect any changes.

You may need to educate people around you. At one point I used to lie in bed at night with my book face down on my chest while I stared into space. Emerging from the bathroom, Rosemary would ask what was wrong. I realised that I hadn't explained what I was doing. I had noticed that I was having difficulty giving the book my full attention and felt that there was probably something unfinished about the day. So I would put the book down and just let my mind wander for a few minutes, returning to the book when I felt ready. Sometimes I would know what the unfinished thing was and sometimes I wouldn't: it was out of conscious awareness. I still do this from time to time and although I've explained it to Rosemary, some part of me still feels that she probably thinks I'm slightly bonkers.

BECOME MORE SENSITIVE AND PAY ATTENTION TO THE DETAILS

As well as paying attention to the 'little voice', you need to raise your awareness of what is going on outside your body, and how it affects you. The details matter more than they appear to. Ignore less and tune in more, since this acuity is your guide as to where to take action. It is like having more sensitive gauges in a car, giving you feedback so that you can spot potential trouble and take corrective action to avoid breaking down.

The good news is that this acuity develops naturally the more you give it attention. Once you start to notice that things do affect your energy, you 'tune in' automatically. It is a little like discovering, after having bought a new car, that virtually every other person is driving the same model. What happened? Did a lot of people really conspire to buy the same car on the same day you got yours, just so that you would feel less special? Possible, but unlikely. More probable is that you are now more aware at a less-than-conscious level and that part of your brain looks out for these phenomena labelled 'interesting car' and keeps telling you each time it comes across one: There's one, there's one, there's another, there's another, etc.

If you wish to accelerate the development of your acuity here is one way to do it. First pick which bit of sensory acuity you want to work on from the following grid. Visual and Auditory refer to using your eyes and ears. Kinaesthetic refers to sensations inside your body – your internal awareness of muscle movement and of feelings. Narrow and broad refer to how tightly focused your attention is spread.

	Internal		External	
	Narrow	Broad	Narrow	Broad
Visual				
Auditory				
Kinaesthetic				

Pick one of the twelve options and then spend 5 minutes at a time considering what you notice in that area. You can start narrow, internal and kinaesthetic, for example thinking about what is going on in your little toe on your left foot – you'll be amazed by how rich a life that digit has. (Try it sometime when you are travelling on public transport.) Or you can go broad, audio and external, and listen for all the noises outside the room. The world and our bodies are always overloaded with sensory information and we normally filter them hugely to make them manageable. We would go nuts if that weren't the case. This exercise is an opportunity to move the filters around a bit.

> There are no little things. Little things are the hinges
> of the universe.
>
> *Fanny Fern*

Notice the details. Little things are the messengers of
the universe. Notice that spark of interest or that damp-
ening of energy. Pay attention to that slight sagging of the
shoulders, the dropping of the head or the long sigh. The
body is eloquent and remarkably sensitive. Sometimes
others can see the changes in our body before we can.
Just how clear these changes can be was illustrated to me
on a training course I attended in Neuro-Linguistic
Programming (NLP). The trainer asked a volunteer to
stand on the stage with her back to the audience. She was
then asked to think of someone she really liked and the
audience was invited to study her posture. Next she was
asked to think of someone she couldn't stand and the
audience was again invited to study her posture. Then she
was asked to think of the person with the shorter hair,
without saying who it was, and the audience had to guess
which person she was thinking of and to call out. She
then told the audience the correct answer, which gave
them the chance to recalibrate.

The exercise was repeated ten times with questions
such as: think of the person you've known longer, lives
closer, is older, etc. Each time the audience would call
out who they thought it was that she was thinking of
and after each set of guesses she would tell them the
answer. This gave the audience several opportunities to
fine-tune their observations, and by the end, most of the

audience was able to get it right most of the time.

If the external changes are that obvious then the internal ones are probably more so – they just need our attention. This requires time and stillness, and that is the challenge – to stop doing and rushing long enough to notice more of what is going on inside.

BE SELFISH (ABOUT SELF-CARE)

The better shape you are in, the more help you can be to others. In order to achieve this you need to become more selfish. This is a precursor to making the rest of the book work.

> Any little bit of experimenting in self-nurturance is very frightening for most of us.
>
> *Julia Cameron*

The idea that you need to be selfish is controversial and, to begin with, causes some people a lot of difficulty. They seem to think that it means trampling over others and thinking only of yourself. This is *not* what it means. It means you need to treat healthy self-care as a priority, as you do when you help someone whose car has a dead battery. Having connected the cables, the advice from experts is that you start your own engine first, before attempting to start theirs. This is so the effort expended in starting theirs will not drain your battery. Similarly, on planes, the safety advice tells you to put your own oxygen mask on first before attending to your children, one reason being that, if you try to help your children first, you may pass out before you are able to do so. In addition, if your needs are taken care of first, then you will feel less anxious and therefore better able to help others.

> When we truly care for ourselves, it becomes possible to care far more profoundly about other people. The more alert and sensitive we are to our own needs, the more loving and generous we can be towards others.
>
> *Eda LeShan*

Self-care works this way – it gives you a sustainable foundation that puts you in a better position to help others. As you take better care of yourself, you can take better care of others. We've all met, or perhaps even been, people who are irritable because they are always trying to meet everyone else's needs but their own.

So why don't we take better care of ourselves naturally? Why do we neglect ourselves and need to be told to take better care of ourselves? Partly it's to do with being criticised when we were growing up for being selfish: we learned it was a bad thing in a global, non-discriminating way. Some of us grew up with the code 'FHB', which stands for Family Hold Back. This was used when guests were descending and there was a chance that there would not be enough food or cake or whatever to go round and we were told to put the guests' needs first. There is an assumption in this view of the world, that the size of the pie is fixed and that if one person is selfish, then others will have less. This is not always true. If someone does exercise to take care of his or her body, it doesn't mean that someone else has to do less. Likewise, if someone has a bubble bath with nice music it doesn't mean that someone else has to go without. What nobody ever taught us when we were growing up is that you can take being selfless too far, that putting yourself last leaves you in a worse position to help others. The criticism of selfishness derives from scarcity-based thinking. The healthy view of self-care is based on abundance-based thinking. Scarcity thinking makes the assumption that there is not enough of whatever to go round and that the only way to get a share is by others going without. Conversely, if you go without, then others will have more. With abundance thinking, the assumption is that there is more than enough to go round and everyone can get their needs met without impacting anyone else.

So how do you start to take better care of yourself? One way is to learn to say 'no'. For such a small word it carries a lot of baggage. We feel guilty when we say 'no', and we are afraid that we become less likeable. Or at work we may be afraid that if we say 'no' we may look as if we 'can't handle it'.

Keep in mind that you are always saying no to something. If it isn't to the apparent, urgent things in our life, it is probably to the more fundamental, highly important things. Even when the urgent is good, the good can keep you from your best, keep you from your unique contribution, if you let it.

Stephen Covey

Many of us find it very hard to say 'no'. One way to do it is to simply not to say 'yes' immediately. Instead, thank whoever for asking then ask them for time to consider, and tell them you will get back to them in a day or so. If they need to know immediately, then the answer is no. That gives you a cooling off period during which you can review your bigger goals and consider whether what you have been asked will get you closer to them or not. Saying 'no' can also command a certain grudging respect from the other party. Most people have a problem saying no and you can act as a positive role model for them. Practise saying no, start with small things and set a goal for the day, for example say 'no' on x number of occasions – you decide how many will be a stretch for you.

Another idea is to consider what aspects of your self-care you may be neglecting. Do you wish you had time to shave your legs or to enjoy a bubble bath? Would you rather wake up to some beautiful music instead of the news, but part of you feels you should be well informed? Or do you wish you had time for a cycle ride at the weekend? Be willing to do a deal to get what you really want. It will cost you, but if it's what you really want it's likely to be worth it. For more on this see Chapter 7, Make Time for Energy Boosters.

You need to treat self-care as a priority in order to raise energy and your biggest tools are to think abundantly and the word 'no'.

BE MORE ASSERTIVE ABOUT WHAT *YOU* WANT

To make these changes work we need to become less 'reasonable' and compliant, less ready to automatically fit in with the wishes of others. That may seem odd and I don't mean we need to be awkward and difficult, but we need to feel less obliged to please others all the time. In particular, we need to run the risk of not fitting in so well with *our idea* of how others want us to be. Beware of the gap between what we think others want and what they tell us directly – it is always worth checking to avoid situations such as: 'I didn't ask because I thought you wouldn't want to.' Be true to what you want and expect some resistance. You may not get any, but don't start with the assumption that the road will be smooth all the way. Hope for the best and plan for the worst.

> The reasonable man adapts himself to the world; the unreasonable one persists in trying to adapt the world to himself. Therefore all progress depends on the unreasonable man.
>
> *George Bernard Shaw*

As you make changes that are good for you, some people will be inspired by this new you, this person who says

what they want and don't want. Others may feel uncomfortable. They may try to bring you down a peg, and
if that doesn't work, they may avoid you. Don't be cal-
lous, but don't let them divert you. You probably only have
one life; make it the one you want. Even if you have more
than one life, make each of them what you want. Please
yourself, and then at least one person will be happy. If you
are within a relationship, I suggest you negotiate this with
your partner, as in the next example.

A friend of mine told me that he had had a really good
holiday with his partner because he had told her exactly
what he most wanted to do and see, and she did the same.
They then both worked out an itinerary that accommo-
dated each other's wishes as much as possible. By asking
for what they wanted and being willing to give more in
order to get it, they both got more. In the past, he might
not have said what he wanted, because he was afraid she
would not be interested and he did not want to make her
do things she didn't want to do. What might previously
have been a conversation they each had in their heads was
made overt this time.

A lot of people have difficulty being assertive, even
senior business people. They get tongue-tied when they
want to communicate something they believe to be
unpopular. This is very understandable. I have two suggestions:

1. Prepare
Before you embark on the conversation, prepare for 5
minutes and write down the answer to the following
question:

> If you were not concerned about their reaction, what would you want to say to them?

People often have difficulty being clear and concise about what their core message was. The advantage of this question is that it allows you to separate yourself from the emotion surrounding the situation and frees you to think at your best. It is often beneficial to use your hands to help you to separate the thinking from the feeling. Start by putting both hands open, palms up, in front of you. Imagine putting the emotion of the situation in one hand, then close it and move it to one side. Then look to the other hand and ask it the question.

Having got clear about the core message you can then bring in the emotional side and ask how you will manage the situation in order to minimise the risk of the reaction you fear and increase the chances of a more positive reaction. Using this technique, I've watched a client rehearsing how he was going to tell one of the people who reported to him, someone he had known for over a decade, that he was seriously under-performing. As part of his preparation, he decided to make the new assumption that their friendship would get even stronger as a consequence. And it worked well – he told him the facts straight and the individual accepted his points.

On another occasion I worked with Christopher, who had to tell his direct report, Joseph, that a newer employee was about to be allocated a significant shareholding in the business in recognition of his greater contribution. My client, Christopher, expected Joseph to be very upset and angry at being seemingly upstaged, and he was not looking forward to delivering the bad news. Formerly, Christopher would have handled the announcement by calling Joseph into his office and telling him he had some news that Joseph might find difficult. He would then have sat back and waited for the inevitable outburst. On this occasion, in order to minimise the risk of upset, he spent time with me planning how to do it differently. He called Joseph in for a meeting, having made sure he had several items on the agenda, one of which was the share allocation. He told Joseph the news in a neutral tone, asked for comment and moved on to the next item. It worked a treat; there was some upset, but slight compared to what he had previously feared, and the relationship is as strong as ever.

Our very fear can turn an unpleasant possibility into a probability. There are, however, tools for avoiding such situations.

2. Make a request
The second suggestion is to use the following sequence, which I have come across on several training courses dealing with assertiveness, when you want to communicate something difficult:

1) When you do _____ (*name the behaviour*)
2) I feel _____ (*name the feeling*)
3) And what I would like is _____ (*make a request*)

Fill in the first blank by naming the behaviour, not the person – there's a big difference. If you talk about the person, they are more likely to defend themselves or counter-attack rather than listen. Talk about what you can see, which is harder to argue with, not what you imagine may be the intention or motives of the person. For example, observations such as, 'when you raise your voice', 'when you start shouting', 'when you interrupt me' are all hard to argue with. They are better than 'when you get angry', 'when you lose it', 'when you act like a five-year-old' or 'when you throw one of your fits', all of which could lead to an argument before you are even able to make the request.

Once you have named the behaviour, move on to what you felt in response. This may be totally new information for the other person. Feelings are not observable and the other person may not know the full effect of their behaviour on you. Although we sometimes think what we feel must be obvious or that the other person should have known or been able to guess what we would feel, this isn't necessarily the case. This sharing of information about your feelings can make a big difference just by itself – often they will say something along the lines of 'Oh, really? I had no idea. That wasn't what I intended.'

The third step distinguishes what you are saying from a complaint about the past. It is a straight request about the future, that they can accept, reject or counter-offer. Again it is concerned about levels of behaviour. You are asking them to *do* something different, not *be* something different. For example:

'When you ask me to empty the bin in that exasperated tone, I imagine you think that whatever I may be doing is not as important as what you are doing and that you feel I should have done it already. That hurts and I feel angry. I would like you to make the request this way in the future: "When you have a moment, please empty the bin." Will you?'

If you prefer, set a time limit: 'When you have a moment, please empty the bin. I'd really like it done before I start dinner. Will you?'

The little question, 'Will you?', is a useful check on commitment. Without it you cannot be sure you have their agreement. It is a powerful question. You can use it in many different situations and it is especially good in business where people sometimes appear to agree but do not commit fully. If you simply make a request and get little or no response, you can't tell if they didn't hear or if they didn't agree. Asking, 'Will you?', and waiting, with full attention, for an answer does take a little longer, but it eliminates the doubt, which saves a potential energy drain later.

'MAKE DO' TO 'CAN DO'

This is an attitude shift: accept that you want things to be different and that it is possible, reasonable and achievable. Shift from 'Make do' to 'Can do'. Accept that getting by, surviving, but barely having enough are no longer good enough and that you deserve better. I frequently meet people who can be very plausible, but boring, when explaining why an often undesirable thing is the way it is. They can give me countless, deadening reasons for having reached this situation, until it begins to feel like it is inevitable and that there is no point in wishing it otherwise. As I listen to them, my metaphoric hand reaches for another drink, or a pistol (to put one of us out of our misery), and my energy sinks. And the reasons always sound important – evolution, the economy, competition, employment procedures, the heritage of a feudal economy, etc.

But however valid the reasons, they can also become excuses for not taking action. Stravinsky, when asked his opinion of music theory, replied: 'hindsight'. The theory did not help him create; it came later to explain what he did. Explanations for the way things are can often make a situation feel more reassuring, but they do not help create change unless they are challenged. Prior to Roger Bannister running the 4-minute mile there were lots of reasons offered by medical experts as to why it was not possible, including the idea that the human body would self-destruct. Had he wanted, there would have been no shortage of reasons for not attempting it. One of Bannister's breakthroughs came from deciding to think of it as improving on a 240-second target. This reduced the size of the challenge and removed some of the negative significance associated with 4 minutes.

> Discovery consists of seeing what everybody has seen and thinking what nobody has thought.
> *Albert Szent-Gyorgyi Nagyrapolt*

Circumstances can seem fixed and immutable until something comes along to challenge and change them. But the reasons for change are often only clear in hindsight. Few of the people paid to spot future trends were able to predict the really big events – Black Monday, the fall of the Berlin Wall, the Gulf War, etc.

You can't create something new just by looking at why things are the way they are. You need to move from 'Why?', which tends to be static and invites defence, to 'How?' or 'Why not?', which have a more dynamic feel. In essence, if there is something you want, don't give up just because you can find reasons to justify why it might be difficult. Putting a man on the moon was one of the defining moments in history, but was not initiated because people thought it might be easy.

The brain seems to respond to questions, particularly facilitating ones. One good example comes from a book called *Rich Dad, Poor Dad* about creating wealth, by Robert Kiyosaki. He suggests that if you want something that initially seems too expensive, you can alter your thinking with a question. Instead of saying 'I can't afford it', ask yourself the question '*How* can I afford it?' If you say the former statement the brain stops thinking, but if you ask the latter question, you engage the brain in problem solving.

A similar transition occurred to me when developing a programme for people who wanted to be truer to themselves, to stop holding back, and be less prone to fit in with how others wanted them to be. Initially, I felt that businesses would not be willing to pay for this, since it felt more like a personal benefit. But then it occurred to me that there was an implicit assumption, untested, that all businesses think the same way. If the reverse were true and all businesses wanted the service then I could not have coped, so the reverse was not a desirable situation either. All I wanted was a few businesses to be interested in it for their employees. Did I think they were out there? The answer, I felt, was yes. That felt much more energising and I then recruited several business people to join the group.

If you think your situation is hopeless, that very thought makes it more so. But the fact that you are reading this book indicates a desire for things to be different, a sense that there is hope. Hang on to that. I once heard someone say:

> A problem is just something you
> want to be different.

What I like about this is that it takes the emotion and blame out of 'problem' and turns it into a more neutral 'situation'. Since a lot of changes are inevitable and healthy, this view can be liberating. It implies: expect changes and expect to want changes. It is nobody's fault, it does not make anybody less of a person, it just needs to be handled. In fact, there is something healthy in wanting a lot of changes – it is the opposite of stagnating.

I was once learning to play the guitar and when I played a piece to my teacher I made a mistake and swore. He looked puzzled and asked me why I swore. It seemed obvious to me, but as he was American and I'm English, maybe it needed explaining. I told him, 'I don't like making mistakes.' He said, 'Oh.' Then he explained that he saw mistakes differently: mistakes just told him where he needed to put in more practice. This was an eye-opener. I used mistakes to beat myself up and he used them to tell him where to put his attention, like a road map for future practice sessions or an agenda for his practice time.

There was no blame or emotion in his view, mistakes were a form of feedback and his view was much healthier. There was no way I was going to learn how to play without some mistakes. If I was going to attach emotion to each of those, then progress was going to be slow and I might even stop because the whole experience was going to be too painful. I loosened up after that.

Most of us would regard walking as a successful means of getting about. However, I read a line from a newspaper feature that described it as 'a series of arrested falls'. When I think of 'falling', I normally think of mistakes or failure, something you don't want. This view redefines falling. It removes the notion of mistake and says that falls, or at least falls in conjunction with arresting, are effective in producing a desired end.

So decide what you want, instead of just getting by, and don't get discouraged by the risk of making mistakes. Treat them as feedback, or as the beginning of something else (like walking) and ask what is to be learned from them. At the very minimum they tell you that you are looking for a different result and this way of going about it produces something unintended. This is not a reason to believe it can't be done, but a reason to believe that another way may be more effective. Edison made over nine thousand 'unsuccessful' light bulbs before he made one work. His view was that none of them were wasted effort since with each he learned a different way to make one that did not work.

> Fall seven times, stand up eight.
> *Japanese Proverb*

NOTICE WHAT DRAINS YOUR ENERGY AND WHAT INCREASES IT

Having increased your sensitivity, the next step is to notice how things affect you and begin to categorise which things drain your energy and which increase it. This includes what you do, who you are with, what you wear, where you are, how you sit or stand, the noise around you, the smells, the sights, etc. Having done this, you need to do less of what drains your energy and more of what boosts it. At one level it is as simple as that. Do more of the stuff that is good for you and less of that which hurts. Sounds obvious, and it is.

'Hhhm, I've always liked this station. This end of the platform suits me better than that. I hate looking at that poster. This button is loose – hope it makes it through the day. I'm pleased to be wearing these shoes today. I really must use the library more.' These are all clues about your energy and what drains and lifts it. In later chapters we will look at more, but you can start now, wherever you are. Put the book down for a moment, take a look around, and notice your reactions to the different things in your environment. Look for little sparks – tiny stirrings that begin to ignite or dampen your aliveness and don't censor. It will speed things up if you can do this with a buddy or partner, since they will notice things that you don't. As you tell them about what went on in the day, they may notice changes in your voice and posture that you miss. As they tell you what they notice, you can choose to pay more attention to them in the future.

TAKE LOTS OF SMALL STEPS

You don't have to do everything in this book all at once, or even ever. You will still get some benefit if you do only one part and take lots of small steps to implement it. The good news is that the effect is cumulative. You take a few steps and the momentum carries you forward. You feel a sense of progress and hope that sustains you to take the next steps. It is a virtuous spiral. But beware – progress is often bumpy, rather than smooth. Whenever we learn something new, the path is rarely a straight line.

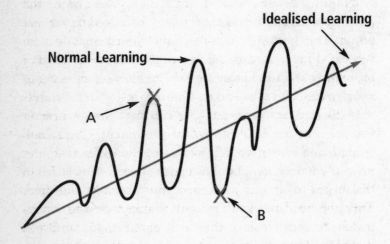

At point B we may be considerably worse than we were at point A in spite of additional time and effort. Do not be harsh on yourself, just allow for it as part of the normal pattern. I temporarily forget even important things I know. I seem to need to keep reminding myself that today can be one of the best days of my life, regardless of what I have got planned. The process starts with making the decision to allow it to be one of the best and to participate fully in whatever I am doing. This is one of those lessons that seem to require frequent re-learning and those spikes of remembering form the shape of my learning curve.

Another possible hurdle to taking lots of steps is that some of us can only handle so much success. Fear of success is almost as common as fear of failure and there seems to be less patience for it. It is a real phenomenon and one that therapists trained in Transactional Analysis (TA) say can trigger a 'script backlash'. This means that if you have a strong internal message telling you that you are not a success and then you start to achieve a measure of it, such as by implementing the material in this book, then there is a risk that a part of you may sabotage progress to slow you down and to somehow keep you consistent to your old beliefs. This has happened to me more than once, at times when I have made progress quickly.

If this happens to you, notice it, accept that it is pretty normal, and seek help from an experienced and qualified therapist. At this time you will need someone who can be objective about your behaviour since you will be in the middle of it and your perceptions may be distorted. Treat the need to see a therapist as akin to seeing a dentist for a tooth that hurts or a plumber to remove a blockage. They all help with problems that reduce the quality of your life and you deserve better. You are not less of a person for seeking timely and appropriate help.

Throughout this process, it is terribly important that you take stock and give yourself credit for the progress you have made. If you fail to do this, future progress will be slower and effort will be wasted since it will not be consolidated. We tend not to do enough of this on the whole. Take the time to notice what you feel, locate where it is in your body and give it a label. If it helps to make it clearer then tell someone else – I have started telling my children when I feel happy and when I am not in a good mood. It seems only fair to alert them to some of the behaviour that may follow. It also helps me connect with my good moods at the time they occur, so that happiness isn't always a product of hindsight.

> What a wonderful life I've had! I only wish I'd realised it sooner.
>
> *Colette*

One structured way to take stock comes from the book *The Inner Game of Work* by Tim Gallwey, who advises us to use the STOP tool. This stands for:

- **S**tep back: put some distance between you and the momentum of your normal life
- **T**hink: gather your thoughts
- **O**rganise: make any course corrections
- **P**roceed: resume

I once used this structure very effectively in one job where I was responsible for coordinating budgets for several departments. In this company, the budget process lasted several months, with a peak in workload towards the end. In the final couple of days before the deadline, I disciplined myself to stop what I was doing *every half hour* for a minute or so, to consider what unexpected changes had happened in the previous half hour: who had not delivered something, who still needed chasing, who had made an amendment, when we expected to get approval for that amendment, etc. Then, if necessary, I would re-prioritise my team's activities for the next half hour. Using this technique meant I had a profound confidence that I knew what was going on, I was clear that the best decisions had been made and I felt an eerie sense of calm in the middle of frenetic activity.

The STOP tool enables us to organise our reviews in order to help us integrate what we have learnt and get the maximum benefit from it. It is something that not many of us do, because we are often so busy moving on to the next thing. So to boost energy, remember to take lots of small steps and STOP long enough to give yourself credit.

TAKE DAILY ACTION (THINKING IS NOT ENOUGH)

> A knowledge of the path cannot be substituted for putting one foot in front of the other.
>
> *M. C. Richards*

You need to deliberately set out to change habits by taking action on a daily basis. You may make some progress through the power of thought alone but progress will be much faster if combined with daily action. And action is easier with focus, structure and support. Be prepared to notice that cause and effect are not always linear, because everything is linked – i.e. make a change in one part of your life and something happens somewhere else.

If you want to establish several new habits produce a daily checklist like the one below, and put it somewhere visible where it can act as a reminder:

	Day 1	2	3	4	5	6	7	8	9	10	etc.
Wash my glasses	✓	✓	✓	✓							
Drink 2 litres of water	✓	✓	✓								
Fix a petty annoyance	✓	✓		✓							
List six things to get done today	✓										
STOP time	✓	✓	✓								
Appreciate someone	✓	✓		✓							
Contact a friend		✓									
Break for lunch		✓	✓								
Read for pleasure	✓		✓								
Tidy for 10 minutes	✓										

Over a period of time, you will quickly be able to see how you get on. If some items seem to be not happening everyday, *please* don't reprimand yourself. Give yourself credit for doing them more often than before. If you don't do them even once, then take them off the list: the time or the item may not be right. And there's no point having them visible if it makes you feels worse – this will just drain energy.

OVER TO YOU

1. Set aside some time each week to review this material. Take your diary or scheduler and, initially, for the next month, put in four slots that work for you that could become regular and routine. Habits are established much more quickly if they are part of a routine. Ideally, you want half an hour a week of STOP time. If you can't manage that, then go for 10 minutes: just the act of putting it in your diary may increase your energy as it will begin to put you in charge and you will feel a difference, particularly if you intend to follow through. In this time you will be reviewing your successes, your learning and identifying the next steps with this material.

2. Think of someone you need to have a mildly difficult conversation with – you can work up to more difficult conversations later. Spend 5 minutes answering the following question and either write the answers down or tell them to a willing partner: 'If I was not concerned about their reaction, what would I want to say to them?'

3. If this is appropriate for you, start saying 'no' three times a day and keep a written record. It is important to write it down in one place and keep a log of your victories – the accumulation of victories makes a difference and speeds up the process of integrating the new behaviour.

4. Build in quiet time to your day – leave the radio

off at home or in the car, don't read a book straightaway on public transport. Allow your mind to
wander. Trust that it usually has something to say
to you.

5. Start paying more attention to which things reduce
your energy and which increase it. Notice where
in your body you feel the reactions. You may begin
to notice how many things affect you that you
were previously ignoring.

Chapter 2

GET RID OF THE LITTLE THINGS THAT ANNOY YOU

Identify those little things that you intend to fix and start sorting them out. It takes energy to ignore them.

If you decide to do only one thing from this book, make it this, since it will give you the most immediate payback for the effort you put in. Some people who have attended my workshops have reported benefits from investing as little as 15 minutes.

What do I mean by 'those little things that annoy you'? Virtually anything that annoys you, such as the things listed below, which were all either suggested by my coaching clients or by people I know:

- a loose or missing button
- shelves that sag with too much stuff
- e-mail backlog
- a dripping tap
- mould around the bath
- light bulbs that need replacing

- things that need to be returned to shops
- odd assortment of things waiting to be glued
- no room in filing cabinet
- drawer that doesn't shut properly
- house not finished
- car breaking down
- garden in poor state
- noise
- double glazing sales people calling in the evening
- committee participation
- weight
- divorce not finalised
- newspapers waiting to be read.

You may have noticed that some of these items are big – I will return to them later. All of them are a drain on energy and create drag. We pick up a lot of drag in our lives; little things that slow us down, which we hardly notice and come to think of just as part of life – inevitable friction, like barnacles on a ship's hull. The good news is we don't have to put up with them and life is different if we do something about them.

Often it is some minor annoyance or irritant that you are tolerating, but are not happy about. Usually you know what to do to fix it, but you have not yet got around to doing it. It does not seem either important enough or serious enough to merit immediate attention, so you put up with it for a while, and sometimes literally years can pass in this way. In the end you sort of *almost* don't notice the loose light fitting, the missing handle, the door catching at the top, the bit of foreign money left lying around from your trip to India eight years ago. You come to accept it; you work around it and it seems like no big deal.

It's not just stuff around the house. Other rich sources include our children's behaviour, our habits, the car, our body, the behaviour of others, the office, colleagues and equipment. As you start to notice these irritants you'll see that they are all over the place and once you tune in, you can list literally dozens. I made a list of things that irritated me about my car: the sun roof was sticking, I wasn't sure the air conditioning was cold enough, there was still sand in the back from our holiday months earlier, the tyre pressure was too high, the aerial was not retracting fully, one door panel was loose, the inside hadn't been cleaned for six months, the outside was dirty – there were eight things just in the car.

Now imagine that all the little jobs around the house requiring attention have a Post-It note attached: the bills say 'pay me', the books say 'read me', the letters say 'reply to me', the stain says 'clean me', the wall says 'paint me', the sofa says 'replace me', the picture says 'straighten me', the papers say 'file me'. That image scares some people, since there could be dozens of these notes in view at any one point in their house. Let's add to it. As you move through the house, imagine each has a nagging, whiny voice saying 'me, me, me!' The voices are all different but all of them are grating. And as you go to make a cup of tea, cook dinner or leave for work, some part of you is engaged in saying, 'later, later, later, not important enough, too busy right now'.

We are so busy that these little things do not seem to justify a high priority. But it takes energy to ignore them. And that is the cost – the energy spent on ignoring them is wasted and it adds up. Imagine paying a day's wages for a bottle of fine wine and, just as you are about to have your first sip, some fly starts buzzing around you, but you carry on drinking. Most people would not be able to enjoy the wine to the fullest and the money spent would be wasted in part. That is how it is with a life that is full of these annoyances. You may still finish the glass but the experience will be diminished. You simply have less available attention to give the wine, because part of you is engaged in ignoring the fly. What makes this trickier is that you get used to these irritations and accept them as inevitable. It is like when turning off the computer you notice the noise of the fan stops and your shoulders drop a little and you sigh. It didn't appear to be bothering you while it was on, but when it goes off you notice that it was taking something out of you.

I once walked into a meeting at my son's future school where the head teacher was talking to a group of parents. I noticed that I found it slightly hard to hear because an extractor fan was on. I wondered if I was being rude or impertinent, but I decided to take the risk and so I went over, studied the controls, found a likely button and turned it off at the first attempt (relieved that I hadn't turned it up). Then I had an anxious moment after the noise stopped as all eyes focused on me (perhaps they had been making something poisonous in the room earlier on and wanted to make extra sure the fumes had fully cleared). The head teacher then turned to me (was he going to ask me what I thought I was doing?) and said, 'Why didn't I think of doing that an hour ago?' I breathed a sigh of relief. He was just like me. He had been putting up with having difficulty speaking, was raising his voice and probably getting irritated. He might even have felt a bit silly by the simplicity of the solution. (I, on the other hand, felt like a hero and was ready for my next assignment.)

Why do we put up with all this, if it makes so little sense? Part of the problem is that as children we were told to compromise, to be grateful, to not make a fuss, to think of others, not just ourselves. Yet when young children want something, or indeed don't want something, they tend to act on it immediately, and with considerable success. The process of socialising moderates these impulses, and in some areas may go too far.

One Person's Story

One of my coaching clients, James, was unaware of the extent to which he was tolerating the behaviour of the person he shared an office with, until I drew his attention to it. The clue for me was non-verbal: he told me that when he got home he always dropped his shoulders and his body flopped in a dramatic way, which he proceeded to demonstrate for me. So I asked him what this gesture meant. It turned out that his colleague continually interrupted James, and tried to talk to him all day long, or so it felt, so James was keeping his shoulders hunched in an effort to either brace himself or create some kind of barrier. He told me that he was unaware of the impact this person had on him, despite the fact that the first thing he usually said to his wife when he got home was, 'And guess what he did today . . .' Once he became aware, he discussed it with his colleague and eventually they parted company.

On one occasion, I was behind on my accounts by some nine months. The task of completing them seemed too daunting and, of course, was getting bigger all the time. I couldn't face it, but it was bothering me and draining my energy every day. As the deadline for filing my tax return loomed, I decided to commit to working on it for just 10 *minutes*. That I felt I could commit to, and at the end of the 10 minutes I was going to give myself the choice to either continue or to stop. A curious thing happened during the 10 minutes – a new thought entered my head, which was: 'Wouldn't it be nice if this were finished?' I did not appear to have had access to that thought before. I suddenly had this desire to get it completed, which made all the difference. The consequence was that I spent a total of about three days on it over the next two weeks and got it finished before going on holiday. So if you have something big and nasty that you are putting off doing, then try taking a small step and see what changes as a consequence.

When you have a lot of little jobs to get done, consider setting aside a budget (one you can afford, not one that will cause you to suffer in a different way) and hiring someone to take care of them in one go. That's what I did with the repairs to my car. I set a budget, made a list of the problems and discussed with the garage which of them they could fix within the budget. Make sure you can afford it and it will give you a flying start.

For some of the irritants you may not find a solution immediately or you may decide to take no action for the time being. That is fine, just write them down, acknowledge they annoy you, and put the list to one side. When you come back to it some time later you may be surprised how some of them seem to have disappeared, as if by themselves. Once you have taken care of these little nuisances you need to take steps to ensure that they do not build up again. Deal with problems quickly and don't let them turn into long-term energy drains. This will be easier when you start with a blank, or virtually blank, slate.

How does it feel to get rid of a petty annoyance? These are comments from people who have done this exercise:

- 'It feels like taking a series of weights off, so I feel lighter.'
- 'I feel more in control and less like I am behind all the time.'
- 'I feel a sense of progress.'
- 'I enjoy what I do more.'
- 'I get more done.'

Little things are sometimes the symptoms of bigger things. Maintain your curiosity and be prepared to deal with all of it. Watch out for any patterns in the things you allow to build up to annoy you. One of my clients never got to the end of his 'To Do' list and noticed that as he moved down it he started to slow down. The first half of his list would be done quickly, the next quarter more slowly and the final quarter even slower. He eventually realised that part of him was afraid of finishing his list. The meaning that he associated with finishing his list was that he would have no more to do and it was only by keeping *busy* (not necessarily productive) that he would generate income. If he were not busy then his income might dry up.

One of my foibles appears to be to postpone the tidying of my desk and office to another day. The reason seems to be that it gives me the illusion of being needed, if only to tidy up. Without that to keep me busy I might begin to wonder what I was going to do, and that can be a bit scary. A desk that is completely empty, when you run your own business, can be unsettling. Of course, now I know this, I postpone tidying it less, but the habit has not disappeared yet.

Even bigger things can be handled if you are honest about what you are tolerating. A good example comes from coach Talane Miedaner:

> My special project was called 'Neat Street'. I was tolerating two big things about living in New York City – the dirty streets and the homelessness. I didn't like the way my block always looked trashy even though it is in a nice residential neighbourhood in midtown Manhattan. I also didn't feel right about the homeless people. I didn't want to give them money because I thought it would go to drugs or alcohol, but I didn't feel right about just walking by either. Then an idea popped into my head: why not ask the homeless people to clean the streets? I was so inspired I went down to the nearest cash machine and as always there was a homeless man with his cup extended. I asked him if he would be interested in working. He said yes. I told him the idea. If he would volunteer to sweep my block on both sides of the street every day, I would ask each resident on that block to give him a $1 a week donation. (This is a city block so there are over 150 people on our

block.) I told him there was no guarantee how much money he would make, but that he had nothing to lose. He showed up on the block the next morning at 7 am, and I gave him a broom and a dustpan. This was the birth of 'Neat Street'. James, the homeless man, ended up being photographed for an article in the *New York Times* and was also on television. He became a regular part of the community, sweeping the block rain or shine, and ended up making enough money to share an apartment with a friend. Now 'Neat Street' has spread to other blocks, and all sorts of organisations have created partnerships with the homeless to provide them work cleaning the streets. Who knows, maybe one day New York will be a remarkable spotless city.

One client told me that he had considered putting his marriage on his list of things he was tolerating, but, at the time, couldn't bring himself to do it as it would mean admitting to himself the trouble he was in. Three years later, his wife initiated a trial separation. Although he was initially devastated, some months later he was able to admit that he had probably not been happy in the marriage for some years. He later came to terms with the situation. He met someone whose company he really enjoyed, which opened the door to seeing the potential of being much happier. He is still going through the messy stage of separation but is much happier about what the future may hold. So even some of the big stuff can be handled. And it starts with honesty about what is so.

OVER TO YOU

1. You will need 20 minutes and a pen for this. Make two lists of all the little things in your life that annoy you: one list for work, if relevant, and one for your personal life. Start noticing more and more how much there is that is not the way you want it to be. You will start to notice more as your sensitivity increases. Add to the list over time.

Work	**Personal**

2. Then pick three easy ones and deal with them within the next week. By 'easy' I mean items where you know all you need to know in order of fix them and which won't take too long. Examples include: sew on a button, clean the car, tighten the screws on a loose table. Notice how it feels. Then keep going. The momentum will build. You will need to come back to this one on a regular basis as you add more and remove more. Expect your sensitivity and awareness to grow. Even if you don't know how to fix something or can't afford to do so, or are reluctant to acknowledge it, write it down. Power comes from writing it down and telling the truth.

3. At the start of meetings, whether at work or when having a coffee with a friend, take a moment to ask: what can I do right now to make us more comfortable? Change the lights, turn down the music, move the blinds, open the window, close the door, rearrange the seating. By making yourself more comfortable you are removing a potential energy drain, that of tolerating discomfort.

POSSIBLE BARRIERS TO IMPLEMENTATION

Implementing the ideas in this book is not always straight-forward, even when the ideas make a lot of sense. If we did straightaway all the things that we know are good for us, we would be a different species. We would all eat healthily, exercise regularly, floss three times a day, avoid smoking and manage our schedules. However, obstacles seem to get in the way. The obstacles are fascinating and infuriating. Some are small, some are big, some are rational and some would probably sound a bit stupid if we said them to anybody else. They are all real, however, in the sense that they have the potential to stop you or slow you down as you begin to move forward. For that reason they need to be taken seriously.

Before you read on, take a moment to consider what might get in the way of your implementing these ideas with enthusiasm. Write them down here:

_____

_____

_____

_____

The following are obstacles that people have raised in relation to implementing the material in this chapter. I hope I have addressed yours below. If not, then I may have answered them or something similar in another chapter. If I haven't, then please check the message board at my website: www.coachingdirectors.com. Feel free to post a question if it hasn't already been addressed and I will do my best to answer it.

- *With this sort of thing, I often start well then slip back into old ways. How can I sustain the focus?*

It takes twenty-one days to establish a new habit. During that time the effort needed will be greater than later. This is the investment phase, needed to get the habit established as a natural part of your routine. This can work for any new habit you want to put into place.

My optician told me that cleaning my glasses with tissues was scratching the plastic lenses, due to the wood fibres in the paper. So I started washing them daily in soap and water and drying them on a towel. At first it was a nuisance and I somewhat resented the time involved at the start of the day. Now, having persisted for a while, I feel uncomfortable at the thought of putting on my glasses without washing them. I have a sense that they are dirty and my mind sends me little reminders to do something about it: ignoring those messages is another unnecessary energy drain. It is as if washing the glasses has become the default behaviour and I am much less aware of the time taken because it is a natural part of my routine, not another 'task' I have to think about fitting in. It is moving closer to the same level as putting on my shoes before going outdoors – minimal thought and no resistance. See Chapter 1 for a format for keeping track of new daily habits.

- *I don't believe these little things drain my energy.*
  Try a few, and then decide. Set aside an hour or two and do several of them altogether. Then stop and reflect: how do you feel about the rest of the day, about yourself? What is your current energy level? How does it compare with before?

- *I don't know which to start with.*
  Pick some items that could be done in an evening or

a few hours. It is useful to feel some progress quickly so you feel motivated to continue.

- *I don't know what to do to handle it; otherwise I would have done it already.*
  It may be a complex task requiring a series of steps, several of which you're not sure about. One way to make progress is to identify the smallest *single* next step you could take to move you forward, even if it is something as simple as looking up the phone number of someone who could help. Then only *after* you have completed that, identify the single next step after that. That alone may feel like progress and help build momentum. It is sometimes difficult and pointless to look too far into the future since things may look different after you have taken the next step, in other words the second and third step after may only become clear after you take the initial step.

Chapter 3

CLEAR THE CLUTTER

Get rid of the clutter in various parts of your life to release energy.

Be careful with this one, since clutter is deceptive and more significant than it looks. Clutter seems to have a disproportionate effect — at some level we feel it shouldn't matter so much, but it does. We see it out of the corner of our eye and silently, and frequently, reprimand ourselves for it.

> The ordinary arts we practise every day at home are of more importance to the soul than their simplicity might suggest.
>
> *Thomas Moore*

Clutter is everywhere in our work space, our home, the garage, the car, the Filofax, the CD storage area, our wallets, handbags and purses, our pockets and, very importantly, in our heads. You will also find it on the computer (ad hoc filing, hoarding, dated items not removed), the 'To Do' list, our finances, our papers and our drawers.

How did it come to be this way? Most of us own too much stuff, a lot of it not much used – and holding on to it locks in energy which could be better used elsewhere. How do you decide what to get rid of? Try these criteria for getting rid of stuff: if it isn't useful or beautiful, move it on (this excludes people, of course) and release the energy that is locked in. If you haven't used it for a year, then it is a candidate for clearing; the year allows for seasonal items such as Christmas decorations.

> Have nothing in your homes that you do not know to be useful and believe to be beautiful.
>
> *William Morris*

Some people object: 'But it is worth something!' What do you do with it when it probably cost you something to acquire and is still usable? If you seriously intend to use it then keep it, but put a time frame on it. With the rest you have four options, you can:

- Sell it.
- Give it to someone who would appreciate it more (my pasta maker went to a single parent mother whose children used it to shred paper – not what I had in mind, but at least I could see it was actively being enjoyed).

- Jumble it or give it to a charity shop.
- Dump it.

Your possessions represent who you *were*; they are a part of your past. You have probably moved on. Take the opportunity to create space for the new you. Give up on scarcity thinking; start thinking abundantly and allow for even better stuff to come into your life. Allow for the possibility that having more space might, in itself, be the better thing.

Getting rid of stuff can be very difficult for some people. One solution is to get help: get a partner, a buddy. One pair of people who wanted to work on this scheduled a day between Christmas and New Year and they phoned each other briefly every hour to maintain momentum to clear their offices.

> Tidied all my papers. Tore up and ruthlessly destroyed much. This is always a great satisfaction.
>
> *Katherine Mansfield*

Another person, who attended one of my seminars, knew she was no good at clearing clutter, but was still keen to get it done. So, remembering the point from Chapter 7 about swapping strengths with other people, she asked a colleague who was very organised to help her clear her office. They agreed that she would reciprocate by helping him think about the future direction of his career. When I met her she showed me that they were partway through and after a day they had removed seven full bin liners and she felt she had a lot more energy.

How do you handle the clutter in your head? The first step is to identify the source or area of clutter and then find an appropriate solution that reduces the draining effect. One solution is to make a long list and then organise the items in logical groups. Getting organised is a way to reduce the sense of clutter and increase energy.

For me, my in-tray used to be a form of mental clutter. I had the in-tray on the corner of my desk and people would drop something in it up to fifteen times a day, often while I was working on something by myself. I would then try to concentrate on the task at hand but a little voice in the back of my head would be wondering what nasty little thing was now ticking in my in-tray. This was a company which valued quick reactions and I was astounded once to find that a fax I sent to my Managing Director (he was in another building) resulted in him phoning me within the half hour to clarify some of the numbers and question my interpretation.

I found the in-tray a distraction from my work since it was not often that something required immediate attention, but it was disrupting my concentration. So I moved my in-tray and put it on to my secretary's desk, which was just outside my door. I then coached her to review the post and if something looked like it needed urgent attention to bring it in straightaway. For the rest she was to write at the top one of the following options:

- Dump
- Delay till some later date
- Delegate to some suggested person in my team
- Do myself and by when, preferably now if it takes less than 5 minutes.

She would bring in this bundle at the end of the day just before she left for home. I would review it alone and add notes, either agreeing with her recommendations or making another. In the morning we would spend 5 minutes reviewing the recommendations together and explain why I had made any changes, so she was in a better position to make suggestions in future. This one change substantially increased my energy and productivity since I was better able to concentrate knowing that someone was keeping an eye on the stuff that mattered; I had the reassurance of knowing that all the urgent stuff had been brought to my attention.

> Out of clutter, find simplicity.
> *Albert Einstein*

OVER TO YOU

Make a list of all the areas of clutter in your life, such as: car, office, garage, living room, cabinet in bathroom, briefcase, tennis bag, purse or wallet, computer, photographs, CDs – be specific, since each of these will become an area to work on and the smaller the area the easier it is to deal with. Then pick one area at a time and allocate 15 minutes to work on it. At the end of 15 minutes you can decide whether to continue or to stop. If you stop, schedule another 15 minutes on another occasion, and so on. Decide when would be a good time to do this and put the time in your diary. Talk to your partner, if appropriate, and do it together – it is more likely to happen.

One client said he and his wife now spend 15 minutes tidying at 10pm each evening. Previously, they were depressed that there was always so much to do. But they have accepted that their aim is improvement, not perfection, and the strategy delivers – they are delighted with the result: the home is more welcoming and they feel more energy when they are there. With children, clearing clutter could be an almost full time job: there is always a piece of Lego or jigsaw where it does not belong. You get a boost of energy if you go for an improvement.

Areas of clutter

1. _____

2. _____

3. _____

4. _____

5. _____

6. _____

7. _____

8. _____

9. _____

10. _____

POSSIBLE BARRIERS TO IMPLEMENTATION

As always, there are challenges to implementing the clearing of clutter. The following are some of the beliefs that may get in the way of your making progress quickly:

- *If I keep things too tidy aren't I a bit too focused on the minutiae? Surely I should have bigger things to worry about. Only a small, anal mind would be putting things away as soon as they've been used.*

  Remember what outcome you want. Don't focus on the barriers. If you want to be more productive, how can you measure that? If you can't measure it objectively, then use a subjective rating out of ten. Both will work, but the former is better. Then give it a try and measure the result against your desired outcome.

  Labels such as 'anal', 'anorak', 'nerd', 'fussy' and 'particular' are to do with how others see us and are often historical, maybe when someone used that name against us or against someone we knew. For example, many of us, when we were growing up, put in a lot of effort to avoid being called 'teacher's pet', but in the world of work it is different and we are often slow to update the rules. If at work you accomplish a lot but don't let the right people know, then you are putting your job at unnecessary risk. Letting others know about your contributions and achievements has become a key work skill. Labels such as the above do not help and just slow us down. Use what works and let that be your criterion for deciding whether you do it again. Focus on the outcome, not the barriers.

  But beware of overdoing it and creating another kind of energy drain. The idea is to make things tidier, so that it reduces the time wasted looking for things, not perfect all the time, otherwise you end up spending more time putting things away and getting them out again.

- *I may need that thing again soon so there's no point putting it away just yet.*
  This is fine if it is for a short time, but the same argument does not apply if a thing has been handily sited but not used for weeks or even months. The point is valid in principle, but take a hard look at the practice. Often I will leave something for weeks, but it is only after I think about it that I realise that I don't really have anywhere to put it. Which means that I haven't finished thinking about where to put it. So it is a form of procrastination disguised as convenience. It is heartwarming to see how often problems that seemed quite difficult yield quickly under the glare of our full attention.

- *I'm no good at clearing clutter.*
  This is an old belief, which does not serve you well. It's time to test it and, if appropriate, update it. Try asking yourself, 'If I were a tidy person, what would I do differently now?' Then start small – just commit to doing it for 5 minutes once a day to begin with. Alternatively, get a buddy to help.

- *I don't want to be that tidy.*
  This raises a deeper point about our behaviour. We are sometimes able to defend our actions without thinking enough about some of the causes or deeper motivations. One of my clients would like to delegate more

often, but can always justify why it is not appropriate. It is tempting to accept her reasons for not delegating specific tasks, but often it is just a defence for some kind of avoidance behaviour. Her real reason for not delegating more often is that she expects others will not like the tasks she delegates, so she is really avoiding the risk of being unpopular. She now sees this, accepts it, and has since asked me to challenge her in this area 'till she squeaks'.

How can you deal with this kind of avoidance behaviour? Firstly, assume that all behaviour is purposeful, even the stuff we don't like. You need first to understand the purpose of the unwanted behaviour, before trying to change it.

Hidden paybacks come in different guises. One of my clients said she wanted to be more organised, specifically she wanted to complete her tax return on time. When I asked her what was positive about not doing it she was puzzled at first. Eventually she laughed as she realised that the real reason for her reluctance was that she felt the regulations that required her to keep her records for six years were ridiculous. Being late with her tax return was her expression of how she felt about it. Once she understood the reason for her resistance and how ineffective her response was, she was able to move forward. Ask yourself what might be positive about clutter for you – keep asking until you connect with an answer that has some resonance for you.

- *Clutter is a sign that I am creative.*
  If it is, then great. Are you willing to try it another way? If you are not, then there may be some hidden

payback. Resistance takes energy. Explore all the things you may risk if you change. Answer these questions in as many ways as you can:

- The positive purpose of clutter for me is . . .
- What I get out of clutter is . . .
- What I would lose without clutter is . . .
- My clutter says . . . about me.

Take your time over this. Allow at least half an hour and return to it on subsequent days. It sometimes happens that your early answers hit a nerve and uncover something new, but more often enlightenment comes a little later and the earlier benefits are more like rationalisations. Once you have exhausted all your answers then ask which is more important than the rest – which is the biggest payoff. Then you need to find a way to honour that benefit with behaviour that is more constructive.

I saw an example of this on a training course when a woman who said she wanted to give up smoking was asked what was positive about it. After some thought, she was able to give over twenty positive benefits for smoking, including:

- It's a way of rebelling against her parents.
- It's a naughty treat.
- It gives her a way of gossiping with colleagues.
- It gives her something to do with her hands when she is nervous etc.

Having compiled this list she was asked whether she

still wanted to give up smoking. She looked at the list and said 'No'. For the first time she appreciated how much she got from smoking at an unconscious level. And her difficulty in giving up demonstrated the power of the unconscious. Her next step would be to look closely at the benefits that were most important to her and find alternative, more constructive, behaviours that met the same needs. Then, once the alternatives were in place, she would be more ready to give up smoking successfully.

- *I think better with a measure of disorganisation.*
  Unlikely but possible. Try it the other way with an open mind, notice what is different and then decide which suits you best, with the benefit of being better informed.

- *It feels sterile, or I imagine it would if I did it.*
  Yes it may, and it may not be for everybody, but if it works, it works, and if it doesn't then at least you've given it a try. Again focus on the outcome, of having more energy, rather than solely on your objections to the means.

- *It is beneath me.*
  Getting rid of clutter is a form of preparation to be more productive. Top athletes do it: before they take part in a race they will often do a lot of boring preparation to get their bodies and minds ready for the event. The event may only last a few seconds, but the preparation can take months or years. We expect to work at peak efficiency every day with minimal preparation of the space around us and with little regard for its effect on us. This means we are either very gifted or mistaken.

- *It will take for ever to clear it all away so there is no point starting.*

  Look for improvement, not perfection. It is sometimes surprising what a difference 10 minutes spent clearing clutter can make. My wife and I used to do something we called a '5-minute blitz' where we moved quickly through the house tidying anything major we saw out of place. Some things will never be perfect. Feel the difference from making a situation better. Sometimes there is a sense of optimism and energy that comes from taking responsibility for your immediate environment in an active way. You can get a huge payback from taking small steps in the right direction, which then puts you on a virtuous spiral, creating momentum for further progress.

- *What clutter? I don't see it.*

  Either you are already very tidy or you are used to it. If it is the former, you can move on to the next chapter. If is the latter, then ask a friend or two to take a look for you. Sometimes it is obvious to them.

- *I've nowhere to put it all.*

  Go to IKEA or somewhere similar for storage solutions or throw stuff out. If you still have a problem, then get help from someone more ruthless than you. Pay them handsomely for their help so that you take it more seriously. The more you pay, the more you value the advice.

- *Even if I cleared it all once, there is no way I would be able to maintain it.*

  Maybe, but often the energy you get from having done it once makes it easier to sustain. Do not get discouraged if you slide backwards occasionally. Progress is bumpy. If babies learning to walk were as easily discouraged and as full of self-criticism about mistakes as adults, then walking would probably be a lot less common. Try adding it to a checklist of daily habits that you wish to establish (see page 40).

Chapter 4

BUILD IN A MARGIN FOR CONTINGENCIES

Build in a margin of time to your commitments in order to reduce stress and increase energy.

We're all very busy trying to cope with the demands and expectations put on us by work, parents, children and friends, as well as our obligations to others and our own ideas about having it all or what happiness and life should be like. The result is that we rarely feel in complete or, occasionally, even partial control. Much of the time we are fully stretched, struggling to stay one step ahead of the next crisis or sorting out the previous one. This is wearing and it drains energy.

Yes, but (I can hear some of you say) *is he going to tell me to take on less? That isn't an option in my life. If that's what he says, then that's it for this book – into the box for the next jumble sale.*

No, this is not about doing less, but there is a paradox here, which will be uncomfortable for some, at least at first.

The solution is to build in a margin for safety; a cushion in case things go wrong, a reserve that you do not need to use but is reassuring to have around. Ever noticed how the car seems happier and more content after you've just filled up? The opposite is being consumed by survival thinking, where you are always fire-fighting, are close to the edge, on the brink of disaster and running on empty. With a low reserve you are holding it together, but only just. Not only does this take a lot of energy, it is not much fun. The cost is usually stress and a nagging sense of feeling behind or of skating on thin ice. There is trouble if one more thing goes wrong: a child falls ill, a plane is delayed or a nanny leaves. One of our nannies failed to show up for work one morning – we later gathered that she had dyed her hair blonde and become a stripper in Greece.

With each problem there is a sense that the whole edifice of your life will crumble. People who live like this are a pain to be around – you feel tense in their presence and they seem to over-react to every little problem. Partly this is because there is so little slack in their life that little problems have big consequences. The dominoes are very close together: when one goes, a lot go.

On one occasion, a client came to my house, having probably set off late. He burst in saying he had 18 miles' worth of fuel left in the car. He drove a Saab which told him how long the remaining fuel would last, based on the way he was currently driving. Since he had a round trip of some 8 miles, he would in all probability make it. He told me that he had been driving really slowly and carefully all the way over to conserve fuel and clearly it was uppermost in his mind when he arrived. He was so worked up that I was beginning to wonder how long it might take him to calm down enough to focus on the coaching agenda and get him out on time – we had only scheduled an hour. I could picture the white knuckles on the steering wheel. Now imagine how different that journey would have been if he had had a full, or even half full, tank. How much more available brain space might there have been on arrival? What other issues might we have moved on to? How much of the stress of that journey did he carry into the rest of the day?

Building in a contingency or a reserve is akin to having some spare capacity – like a reserve fuel tank or more than enough fuel to comfortably complete a journey so that fuel is not on your mind. With enough 'extra' fuel you are releasing energy for other uses. You still complete the journey but at a lower emotional cost.

When you have a margin for comfort you attract better things into your life than when you are needy. The people who tend to get the most freebies (complimentary tickets, free gifts, hospitality) are those who can most afford to pay. Those who can obtain loans most easily are those who least need them. They can also afford to pay more and yet are in the best position to buy larger pack sizes to take advantage of economies of scale.

What are the symptoms of someone running on empty? Do you recognise any of the following in yourself or in people around you:

- low resilience
- quick to anger, ready to snap
- interrupting oneself and others
- talking too loud

- complaining
- looking strained, close to breaking point
- no fun to be around, no sense of humour
- sarcasm

What are the main causes?

- too much to do
- too many demands and commitments
- too many meetings
- unrealistic deadlines
- too much travel
- saying yes too readily
- neglecting self-care.

What are the consequences? Running on empty impacts on quality of work, stress, home life, attitude to work, colleagues and clients – we've all heard people joke that things would be fine if it weren't for the clients and of junior employees being secretly relieved they did not win a piece of new business.

One of my friends was Marketing Director at a big multinational company based in London. She could see her department through the glass wall and she noticed a pattern. At the start of the day people would move around at a civilised pace, but, as the day wore on, the pace would quicken and the level of noise went up. She realised that the problems began after people had started their first meeting of the day. Often it overran so the next meeting started late. This would get gradually worse until towards the end of the day they might be behind by one, two or even three meetings with people backed up waiting to see them and presumably with knock-on consequences for meetings that the 'waitees' had arranged with others. They regularly underestimated how long meetings took and the consequence was frustration for lots of people. It encouraged an atmosphere of stress.

How do you get out of it? A word of caution first – these ideas are not going to work for everybody all the time. So do not reject them if you can't immediately see how they might apply to you. Modify them to suit your life and look for opportunities to use them where you can, since even partial implementation will help you feel more energetic.

1. *Underpromise and overdeliver*
   Build in some time for things to go wrong. When accepting a request or project and discussing timing, try, where possible, to build in some reserve. Many of us will have been in a position where we have been asked how long something will take. We want to help, to look good, or we might be keen to get the business, so we've said the earliest date it could *conceivably* be done, having taken into account working evenings and part of the weekend and persuading others to do the same. Only later do we find out that the recipient will be on holiday that week or that the first time they will realistically be able to discuss it will be at the board meeting after the next one. If you are asked to distribute some leaflets for your church or sports club, ask when they are needed – do not assume that you have to do it in the first bit of available time you have. Check when things are needed to avoid putting unnecessary pressure on yourself.

It is not always possible to negotiate more than the minimum time but sometimes it is. Look for those opportunities. Allow time for things to go wrong, so if someone else does not do their bit in time, or something else urgent comes up, you can still deliver on time. If all goes well, you may even deliver early.

Imagine a situation where you order something important to be delivered to your house and it arrives on a Thursday. How would you feel if you had been told to expect it on Wednesday? And how differently would you feel if you had been told to expect it on Friday? The actual date of delivery is exactly the same, but managing the expectation makes all the difference in the world.

2. *Be early for meetings*
I used to collect someone en route to an aerobics class. One day I was a few minutes early, so I turned off the engine and sat and waited in the car. When he came out, he rushed over, checked his watch, asked how long I had been there, why hadn't I knocked and generally looked flustered and apologetic. I told him that I was fine and had used the time to review my day and realised that I had had a better day than I had thought. He clearly timed things to within a minute. I used to do this a lot and I remember that I spent more of my time checking my watch rather than doing anything more noble or useful. I used to stand in a pub with my friends till 2 minutes before my train was due, knowing that I could run to the station in a minute and a half and still make it. But I was not good company for those last minutes.

So show up to airports, stations and school early. Show up to meetings 5 minutes early and, if you need to travel, allow an extra 15 minutes and put your departure time in your diary and treat it as fixed as a meeting. You will feel differently en route and potentially differently the rest of the day. And if you show up early, take the opportunity to metaphorically rise up into the air and take a helicopter view and review your day, project or life. If someone else is also early, you can practise your skills at deepening relationships with small amounts of time. Set yourself a challenge of getting a sparkle in their eye – be playful and feel more alive.

I was hilariously early to a meeting with my publishers and while waiting I got chatting with this charming woman who told me some amazing stories about her amateur healing powers. Her mother had been pronounced dead in hospital, but when she turned up and starting massaging her feet, her mother woke up and said: 'Oh hello, Pam.' The doctors looked on open-mouthed. She claims to have saved her husband's life on three occasions. She added to the richness of my day. As well as being early, I was also willing to make contact – see Chapter 5

3. *Build a margin into your meeting times*
If there are only two of you meeting and you are reliant on public transport, or if the traffic is unpredictable, then tell them that you will be there *around* 2pm or whatever time you agree. And check if they are ok with you being a few minutes either side of 2pm. This gives them a chance to allow for a potential delay and

warns them not to put the next meeting too close to the planned end time of your meeting. It also lets you off the hook, reducing anxiety ahead of, and on, the journey.

4. *Be realistic about meeting length*
Allow longer for meetings than the absolute minimum they might conceivably take if everything goes well. I know one person who implemented this and he started to allow an hour for something that previously he would only have allowed 45 minutes for. In his old way of working, he used to try to rush the meeting so that he could finish in 30 minutes, saving 15 minutes to do something else. His staff accused him of listening with his watch. The new approach had two benefits: the first was that he didn't rush so much and, curiously, the meetings went quicker, so that he finished in under an hour, but with less anxiety about the time. The second benefit was that he had fewer back-to-back meetings in his diary – he usually had some space between meetings even if the diary did not look that way. That meant he could draw breath and the next meeting went more quickly too.

It is useful for energy purposes to agree on the length of the meeting. If, for example, you are on a committee to organise a community event, then one of the first items on the agenda could be how long the meeting will last and what the plans are for completing discussions that are not finished in the time allowed. This will align expectations and reduce the potential energy drain experienced by people wondering what time they will get away and what might happen if their part of the agenda does not get enough time.

5. *'Keep-free' time*
    One client has a 'keep-free' half-day each week to tidy up or catch up on stuff not done earlier. He has briefed his secretary that she is allowed to move the 'keep-free' slot in order to put in a meeting but only if there is somewhere else *that week* for the 'keep-free' slot to go: he will not allow it to be cancelled. The effect on him is to reduce his sense of feeling out of control.
    One interesting incident happened after a year-end. The client used to rate his own performance each week and e-mailed me about the areas where he wanted to change his behaviour – for example, 'to stop interrupting others', 'listen with undivided attention', 'stop saying how I would do things', 'appreciate support staff'. Several weeks into the new year, he noticed that his self-assessments were getting worse. He then realised that the deterioration had occurred after the start of the new year and became aware that his automatic scheduler had stopped putting the 'keep-free' time in his diary. The consequence was the gradual re-emergence of old habits.

6. *Build in some thinking time each week*
    The ideal is an hour a day, but, if this is too much, then I suggest you start with 15 minutes twice a week. What you do is sit with a notepad and pen with no interruptions and jot down any thoughts that arise. Creating some quiet space enables you to get in touch with your intuition more and allows the thoughts that

often get drowned out by the noise of daily life more chance to be heard. This quiet time will also help you to organise your thoughts and will thus make you more productive the rest of the day.

7. *Notice patterns of lateness*
   I noticed that I used to be *almost* late for many meetings. Almost but not quite. The pattern was that I would leave what seemed like enough time to get ready and travel, but something would always crop up. I then spent the journey wondering whether I would be late, and if so how late, and what excuse I would use and what tone of voice I would say it in. With the help of my therapist, I learned that this anxiety about being late was preventing me from planning for the meeting en route, and from arriving in a composed state of mind. Some part of me wanted this: it kept me from being too successful and thus attracting the envy of people I grew up with. Once I understood that, I started leaving a bigger margin for journeys and now feel much more composed when I get there. I am also able to relax about possible envy now I understand better the source of the behaviour.

OVER TO YOU

Pick which ideas you will implement and, where appropriate, put them in your diary. Treat thinking time as seriously as you would a meeting with someone else. Put in your diary the time you will set off for meetings. Even if you're not convinced by any of this, I suggest you do it anyway – you may just find that it works.

POSSIBLE BARRIERS TO IMPLEMENTATION

- *This will take time, not make it. It will increase stress.*
  Try it and review. There is no need to commit to doing this for ever. Only use it if it works for you, but try it before you decide.

- *Sounds good in an ideal world. Not practical in my life.*
  Work with a friend or a coach to find a solution. You may feel too close to the problems to be able to see clearly and another person may be able to help create some detachment so you can get a better view.

- *Who has time for margins? I don't even have time for the urgent. I'll think about it when I'm less busy.*
  You are right, there is paradox here. However, as you build in margins you end up creating a sense of more time. You will probably need to do it to be convinced. Just start with a commitment to show up to meetings 5 minutes early for one week and see how you feel.

- *Others are in control of my time – I don't have any choice.*
  Untrue! You always have a choice, but you may be feeling so run down at the moment that this is how it genuinely feels. If you are serious about changing it then get help, in the form of a good friend or coach, and soon.

- *My life's a mess. It's too late.*
  Not true! Start now. It's only too late when you're dead.

Chapter 5

IDENTIFY YOUR NATURAL GIFTS

Increase energy by becoming very clear about what your strengths are.

Do you know what your strengths are? What you are good at? We often enjoy doing the things we are good at, but tend to downplay our strengths. We have a tendency to take too lightly the things we do well and to hanker after that which we see others do well. So if we can cook, drive, hit a topspin backhand, balance a chequebook, set up a spreadsheet, then we tend to assume that everyone else can too. When we come across someone who can't, then we tend to assume that maybe the skill can't be all that valuable or difficult. It's sort of charming in a self-deprecating way, but it reduces our energy.

The greatest good you can do for another is not just to share your riches but reveal to him his own.

Benjamin Disraeli

One Person's Story

A friend of mine was a producer of award-winning films and documentaries, but he got fed up trying to get projects off the ground and bringing them to a successful conclusion without compromising on his original vision. He then spent a couple of very unhappy years looking for a job that could use his considerable talents. He had started his career as a copywriter in a successful advertising agency, where he was told, more than once, that he was good, and he knows that he was told in such a way that people were trying to tell him that his was a rare talent. But for him, it was too easy. He left to find more of a challenge. He did not value sufficiently what he had. Last I heard, he was doing two jobs part-time, hoping one of them would become full-time, but neither used his talents to the full. Despite being told clearly that he had a significant talent he didn't appreciate it fully. Had he done so, he might either have stayed and tried to increase the level of challenge within the role, or moved on to something which continued to use this talent while challenging him in other ways.

I came across another illustration of this on a training course on communication skills. The facilitator told a group that most people assume that others are more accomplished than they are. There were a lot of protests from the participants, who told her they did not believe it, so she set out to prove it to them. She asked them to all close their eyes and for the one who thought they were the least accomplished person in the room to put up his or her hand. She then asked the person with their hand up to keep it up and everyone to open their eyes. Everyone had his or her hand up.

Eventually, all attention turned to one particular person, who was asked by the others: 'Why do *you* have your hand up? You're clever. You are very successful, travelling the globe, working on high visibility projects with senior people. You have a big car, big office and a big house.' He told the group that, yes, he had all of those things *but* he could not operate the key to unlock his front door, he could not put together a shopping list, he could not shop at the supermarket and he could not cook a meal.

He gave a lot of weight to the things he could not do which he could see that others were able to do easily. Many of us do the same to a lesser extent. Other people seem more talented. When we see others who have a better memory or are better at engaging with children or doing DIY, we measure ourselves by our weaknesses compared to them. It's a problem-focused approach – the half empty glass. It doesn't have to be this way, nor does it serve us well if it is, for at least two reasons:

1. We lose the opportunity to get energy and enhanced self-esteem from engaging in our strengths.
2. We deny the world the benefit of our strengths (more on this in the next chapter).

So how do we get clear about our strengths? One clue lies in the fact that others can see our gifts more readily than we can – we took them for granted a long time ago.

A lot of schooling is about drawing attention to our short-comings rather than our strengths and talents. So if you got nine out of ten on a test, most of the attention would be on the mistake, not on the fact that 90 per cent was correct. This still works with adults. When I am giving feedback from colleagues on a person's strengths and weaknesses (or development opportunities) they are usually dismissive of the strengths section and want to get on to what they think of as the 'meat' of the feedback. It's all I can do to slow them down to listen to the strengths, which they almost treat as if they are not true, as if they were included to be polite, to add some kind of balance, whereas in truth the strengths identified are always significant and key differentiators between them and their colleagues.

So how, in the absence of hiring someone to do it for you, do you find out how others see you? One solution is to ask other people: 'What is my greatest strength and greatest weakness?' Pick five people, either in a work context or outside or both, and tell them you are doing an exercise that you would like their help with. Pick the people with some care. They do not need to be people who have known you a long time, but you probably need to have a reasonably comfortable relationship with them. When you get the results back, talk them over with someone you trust, to make sense of it all.

When you ask your five for your strengths and weaknesses, give them time to respond – one busy person received this request by e-mail and said she paced her office for half an hour thinking about it. When you get the feedback, do not argue with them, just listen and ask clarifying questions only if necessary. Your job at this stage is simply to seek to understand how they see things from their perspective. Resist the urge to make comments such as, 'You call that a strength!', 'I'm not surprised *you* see that as a strength', or 'And is that the best you can come up with?'

When I ask people to do this exercise they often ask whether they will get the truth. The answer, for the most part, is yes – mostly, the people who receive the request recognise that you are making yourself unusually vulnerable in asking for such personal feedback and they tend to treat the task responsibly. This request invites contact at a deeper level than usual and can take some people by surprise, so it is worth taking a little time to prepare them for the request. Tell them some or all of the following:

- You have a favour to ask them.
- You are reading a book on increasing energy and this is one of the assignments.
- You are making a request of five special people and you have picked them to be one of the five.
- This will help you get a clearer picture of yourself.

Not everyone is comfortable with asking or talking about weaknesses. 'Weakness' is not intended as a negative in this context – it is just another description of an attribute that in some places would be an asset and in others a liability. In asking for weaknesses you get more information about your strengths. Depending on context, the same attribute may be described as:

- creative *or* easily distracted
- focused *or* pig-headed

- confident *or* insensitive
- funny *or* flippant

> What is a strength in one context may be a weakness in another. I'm persevering – you are stubborn. I'm flexible – you are weak . . .
>
> *Malcolm Forbes*

Asking for weaknesses is just another route to identifying strengths – by looking at the other side of weaknesses you have one more opportunity to understand more about something that could be a strength.

OVER TO YOU

Write below a list of five people you feel you can ask. Some people like to ask five work colleagues, plus five friends or acquaintances outside. Plan how much preparation each will need before you make the request, and then decide whether you will do it by phone, e-mail, face-to-face or some other way. Then do it. When you get the results, talk them over with someone you trust, to make sense of it all. It is important to do this, because their objectivity can be very useful in case you feel tempted to dismiss any of the strengths. Once you have done this, move on to the next chapter, which discusses how to maximise your strengths and deal with your weaknesses.

Personal	**Work**
_____	_____
_____	_____
_____	_____
_____	_____
_____	_____

POSSIBLE BARRIERS TO IMPLEMENTATION

- *I don't know five people I could ask*
  We all know at least five people. The personal nature
  of the request may be getting in the way, in which case
  treat this as an opportunity to deepen relationships by
  picking people with whom you'd like to have a closer
  relationship. Some may ask you to reciprocate, which
  will create an extra bond.

- *I'd be embarrassed*
  You're on a journey to a more energetic version of
  you. Isn't the risk of a little embarrassment worth it?
  Embarrassment implies you should not be asking for
  some reason. Why not? Might they think you a bit
  weird or needy to want this kind of feedback or reassurance? I felt exactly the same way when I was doing
  a course to raise my self-esteem. One of my assignments was to call two old friends, tell them I was doing
  a course to raise self-esteem, and then ask them what,
  specifically, they liked about me. I felt embarrassed to
  admit I had a problem with self-esteem and needed
  help. Their reaction was beautiful, they both said

spontaneously that they admired me for doing something about it.

People seem to know, when asked appropriately, that with a question like this you are asking something from the heart and they treat it accordingly. Often they feel privileged to be asked.

- *They'll be nice to me and won't tell me what they really think.*
  It is true that they will probably not want to hurt your feelings. So they may not tell you the absolute worst weakness or they may water it down a little. But they know you would not be doing this if you didn't want the truth. Whatever they do tell you will still be significant and useful.

- *It's too personal.*
  This probably indicates some fear. Ask yourself: what is the worst that could happen? The answer is likely to be a theme in other parts of your life. Treat this as an opportunity to stretch your comfort zone.

- *It takes too much of another person's time*
  It need only take a few minutes, but if they want to spend longer, let that be their choice.

Chapter 6

CHOOSE TASKS
THAT USE YOUR GIFTS

*Look for opportunities to use your strengths even more
and get help to deal with your weaknesses.*

You may have been surprised by some of the feedback
you got from doing the exercise in the last chapter. Now
you know more about your strengths, as seen by others.
It is likely that you feel you have other strengths that
people have not mentioned.

One way to add to your list is to analyse your day.
Make a list as you go through the day, or at the end of
the day, of the things you did that you enjoyed and the
things you did not enjoy. As you do it, make sure that you
suspend judgement, just be a neutral observer. So if you
happened to enjoy writing a funny or thoughtful e-mail
to a friend, or putting a label on a file, then make a note
of that, without judging whether it is important or useful
in some way. You can further add to this list by reviewing
your past career and noting what you enjoyed and what
you did not. Look for the little sparks, those moments that
ignited your feeling of aliveness.

<u>Things I enjoy</u>	<u>Things I hate</u>
GETTING THE FACTS TOGETHER	WRITING REPORTS
LIAISING WITH OTHER DEPARTMENTS	
SOLVING PROBLEMS	IMPLEMENTING SOLUTIONS
PREPARING PRESENTATIONS	PRESENTING TO THE BOARD
COOKING	SHOPPING
DECIDING WHAT TO COOK	WRITING THE SHOPPING LIST
	CHOPPING INGREDIENTS
IRONING	WASHING
WASHING UP	PUTTING THINGS AWAY

Now look at the individual components. It may be that you enjoy one aspect and not another – put the parts in two columns, for example, list that you enjoy setting up projects in one column but that you don't enjoy running them in the other, that you enjoy cooking, but not preparing or shopping, and so on. Start by being honest.   Beware of any limiting assumptions such as, 'What use is gathering information if you are not interested in doing the analysis? Who is going to pay you to just gather information?' Such a statement is not only limiting, but could interfere with the observation. At this stage it is best to assume as little as possible and just acknowledge what you notice. It may be in this example that the enjoyable part of gathering information is actually talking to the people who have the information, so a strength might be interpersonal relations or influencing or negotiation, not necessarily gathering information. Remain openly curious at this stage.

What if you're not enjoying anything? Or if you don't know whether you enjoy something or not. Then something may be going on internally that is getting in the way of your being clear about things, or you may need to raise acuity, to become more sensitive and aware. Take time to notice, and pay more attention to the internal responses to what you are doing. All this takes is time and attention, and the time involved need only be a few minutes. As an example, I worked with a client who wanted to develop a better rapport with his colleagues. I asked what signals his body gave him when he had good rapport. At first, he did not know and resisted the line of questioning, so I left it. Two weeks later, he told me that he had identified a kind of buzzing around his chest area when he felt good rapport. Two weeks after that he came back with another sign – moisture in his eyes. By giving it his attention, he moved from resistance to tuning in. This kind of discovery is wonderful, and makes you realise how much else is going on that we don't pay attention to. For more on how to raise awareness, see Chapter 1.

To get the most value from this exercise don't censor what you enjoy. My wife is an 'executive' who works for a company in market research. What she really enjoys is sorting out and organising projects, i.e. administration and developing systems to make things work more smoothly. However, at one time, she felt that this was not a very intellectual skill and that she should not be trying to make the most of it, especially as it was a company that values intellect. That changed when she switched jobs to a department that was a mess and needed a lot of organising to make it work better. She is now in her element and happy to own her skill.

Be open to change. I used to hate doing the washing-up, with a passion. Rosemary used to say that she could almost see a black cloud over me after half an hour at the sink. I'd be grumpy and in a bad mood for hours afterwards. That was some years ago. Recently our dishwasher broke down. We were without the machine for ten days, and I was doing the washing-up by hand. During this time it occurred to me that I was finding it therapeutic and satisfying. I don't understand it, but there was something fulfilling about washing the lot, not just the bits that didn't belong in the dishwasher, and I was somewhat sad when the new machine arrived. A huge shift for me. So be prepared for things to have changed and look afresh at your likes and dislikes. You do not have to be consistent.

One Person's Story

What we enjoy is an individual matter. One person told me that if he had what he called 'a dirty job', such as fixing cabling, arranging a teleconference or fixing a software problem, he would do it. He did not like to ask others to do things he found unpleasant. Since he was the Managing Director, we both agreed that this was probably not the best use of his time. He has since learned that other people are not the same as him – they may enjoy what he hates – and he now delegates much more happily and is delighted to find people doing jobs he dislikes with enthusiasm. He still can't quite believe that his receptionist seems to enjoy setting up conference calls for him.

I used to regularly lose sight of what I enjoyed by being busy. In my marketing role, I would sometimes be asked if I would be willing to do training of store staff. I would look at my diary, and since it was weeks away and the diary looked OK, I would say 'yes'. Then, two days before the training, I would look again at my diary and at my workload and decide that I didn't have the time. So I would look through the glass wall of my office and look out on my department and choose some innocent member of my team, who had the misfortune to be in at the time and did not look particularly busy, to stand in for me. The irony was that it was only after the job came to a close that I realised that developing people is one of the things that gives me energy. It made me wonder how many other things I gave up or did not notice because I was too busy. So please take the opportunity to learn from my mistake.

Having identified your strengths you need to use them: these are your gifts and the world is a richer place for them. You need to own what you are good at and the more you use them, the higher your energy level will be. This is contrary to conventional wisdom, which says that if you are good at something, then you can afford to neg-lect it, and if you are bad at something then you need to put more effort into getting better. Chances are that if you put a lot of effort into something you are not good at, then you might, after some struggle and energy loss, become average. But if you put the same effort into some-thing that you are already good at you could become world class. It's worth remembering that the people who have a reputation tend, for the most part, to be known, not as all-rounders, but as specialists who excel in one, or a small number of things.

Use your strengths whenever you can. When I joined Coach U, a distance learning course for coaching skills, I was sent over 2600 pages of material, none of which was in order. The first challenge was to organise it into ring binders. A colleague who had also received the material called me and asked if I would like some help to get it organised. I was taken aback by the offer. Why would someone offer to do something so horrible for someone she hardly knew? I said yes, quickly, while trying not to sound too keen, and hurried across with my folders. Once I was there she took the first folder and went through it, identifying what belonged where and what was in the wrong place and compared each section with her own folders. She sorted out my folders in what seemed like no time and at the same time we networked and made use of the opportunity to get to know each other better. She was using a strength, and for her it was not an effort, it was enjoyable.

So who does the stuff you don't want to do? Can you just ignore the tax return and the paperwork? Probably not. The ideal it to find someone else whose strengths complement your own. I used to find it a drag to do the department's monthly forecasts of expenditure, even though I knew it was important for me to be intimately acquainted with it. So I delegated it to someone in my team who was a wizard with numbers and for whom this was no effort. My role became to review what she had done. And afterwards I kicked myself for not thinking of it sooner.

As you consider who can help with the things you don't like to do, remember that people are remarkably different – we sometimes forget how different. Some of these differences show up in our preferences for particular tasks. Some people are people-oriented; others prefer paperwork. Some like big picture stuff; others prefer the detail.

Some have a preference for words, others for numbers. Some are good at creating things, while others are better at finishing them. Some prefer to process visually, others have auditory or kinaesthetic skills.

But you may not be able to offload much of it in the short term. If you can't delegate something to one of your team, perhaps you can hire someone to do that task for you. For example, it seems to take me for ever to get round to sending articles to people who I think might enjoy them and also to send out newsletters. So I have hired a 'virtual assistant' – someone who works remotely and is paid by the hour for what they do. She does some of the stuff that I find I don't get round to quickly. And it works. So the stuff I don't like to do gets done by someone else who I pay less than I charge my clients. This leaves me free to do more of the stuff I actually enjoy, which means I have more energy, so am more productive and profitable.

What can you do if you don't have the option of delegating or buying in support? One course of action is to swap skills with someone who is good at doing what you are bad at. I hate doing my accounts but my wife enjoys it. She is the daughter of an accountant and the process of starting with scrappy little pieces of paper, creating some order and then reconciling them with a bank statement brings her a sense of satisfaction that I can only marvel at. In Chapter 3, Clear the Clutter, I have already mentioned the person who swapped his career counselling skills for his colleague's organising skills. They each swapped a weakness for a strength in a win/win exchange. We can all be equally creative.

Another option for dealing with a weakness is to get

support from a fellow sufferer. I used to be bad at setting goals for the day. So I asked a colleague if she was interested in creating mutual support on this and she agreed. She was also bad at it, but together we were better. We set up an arrangement where we would have a 5-minute phone conversation at the start of the day outlining the three key goals each of us had set for the day. At the end of the day we would talk again to either confess or celebrate. And we also took a moment to summarise what we had learned. To get ready for each of those phone calls, we had to do the preparation that previously we were avoiding, and the system worked well.

The key point is to use what flexibility you have, to think creatively about the kind of solution you would like and not be hampered either by the fact that it has not been done before or by whether or not the other person is likely to agree. At times, I have kept a mental shopping list at the back of my mind, looking for people to join me or support me in some way to get me through things I was not good at. Then, when I found someone I liked the look of, I would tell him or her what I was looking for and see if they volunteered.

But what do you do if none of the above options is available to you, for whatever reason? You may be working in a very competitive culture, somewhere where it would be unwise to show that you have a weakness. Or maybe it would make you vulnerable to talk about not enjoying something that is meant to be part of your job, since someone might just decide it would be amusing to give you more of it. I am sorry to say those people exist. What do you do then?

Firstly, you need to be very clear about what you do

enjoy. Secondly, see how much of what you are currently doing you enjoy, and then decide how much more you would like to do. Thirdly, look for opportunities to do more. You may have to volunteer for projects, or let your boss and others know what kind of opportunity you're looking for. You may have to educate people around you. Expect to have to work, persuade and cajole to do more.

There will be many who will say it is not realistic, that it will not pay, or will offer some other rational-sounding reason to stop you doing what you enjoy. Your enjoyment of what you do may be unsettling for them, bringing into question what they are doing, when previously they were resigned to a job they endured. So be prepared: for some people the fact that you are doing more of what you enjoy will make their lives look less attractive and they may not thank you for that. As a result, they may also not want to support you in your endeavour. Do not let them discourage you.

In one job (which I describe in greater detail in Chapter 10), I decided that I enjoyed my work best when I was being proactive, and then made changes in my priorities to allow me to do that. I decided what being proactive would look like in a concrete way and dealt with some significant obstacles on the way. In this instance I had to educate my boss, my secretary and my team to work together to allow me to do more of what I enjoyed. And interestingly, profits improved also. This was a case of making full use of the flexibility I had. I managed to align my goals and interests with what I knew the company valued, but I did it my way, so that it fed my interests, while making more money for the business.

How can you make fuller use of the flexibility you have

to do more of what you enjoy? If your first answer is that you can't, then I suspect you may be heading for that category of people described as 'comfortably resigned'. And I imagine you may have made the assumption, without having tested it, that it can't be done. In which case you need to do some more thinking. Bear in mind that the clearer you are about what you enjoy, the easier it is to get through the rest of it.

One person I worked with had a long 'To Do' list that was getting in the way of his proactive work, which was needed to develop his new business. He felt weighed down by his list and resented it. But instead of abandoning it, he reframed the way he looked at it, and saw it as a gateway – the sooner he could clear it, the sooner he could do what he really wanted. With that, he stopped resenting it and got on with it and finished it in record time. This is a case of looking forward to something you enjoy and using that carrot to finish what you are currently doing.

OVER TO YOU

Write down in the spaces below the things you enjoy and the things you hate doing. Add to the list by reviewing not only your day, but also your earlier life and career. What is it you really enjoy doing? You may want to do a separate list for work and home. How can you get rid of some of the stuff that gets in the way of you doing more of what you enjoy? Then get support for the areas in which you are weak, and look to expand the areas you enjoy.

Some people hire a cleaner or book-keeper, others hire someone to do the ironing, dusting, to cut the grass or do the decorating. Feel free to be as specific as you want – don't be limited by existing roles or trades. Some pay with money, others swap skills. Ask your partner or friends what they would like from you; it may give you another insight into what they see as your strengths.

Things I enjoy	Things I hate
_____	_____
_____	_____
_____	_____
_____	_____
_____	_____
_____	_____
_____	_____
_____	_____
_____	_____
_____	_____
_____	_____
_____	_____

POSSIBLE BARRIERS TO IMPLEMENTATION

- *No one's going to want to do the stuff I hate.*
  This is probably an untested assumption and one that

holds you back. Suspend judgment, and just make a list of all the things you dislike, then start looking to see who might be able to help, or who might know someone who can help. Then ask *them* what would make it attractive for them: they may be able to see your strengths more clearly than you.

- *This is not the real world — it's pie in the sky.*
  It's worked for others. It's also the basis of successful teams where one team member's strength will complement the weakness of another, and vice versa. What might be different in your life if it worked for you? If that is attractive, then go for it and don't let the difficulties you can see get in the way of starting.

- *I don't have any skills to swap.*
  Ask others what skills you have that they would like to have (for more on this, see the previous chapter). Then believe what they say.

- *I don't have time. I'm too busy.*
  Put this book down and come back when you are ready to take yourself seriously.

- *In this life you have to make the best of what you've got. No one's going to help you. They have enough on their plate.*
  Another untested assumption. When you do find someone with whom you are able to swap skills, you will lighten their load and vice versa. Both of you will effectively have less to do because you're playing to your mutual strengths. Rosemary can do the washing-up faster than I can and I can put up shelves faster than she can. She can reconcile a bank account faster than me, while I can bathe the children faster.

Chapter 7

MAKE TIME FOR ENERGY BOOSTERS

*Make time to do the things that boost your energy –
they will help you through the rest.*

What do you like to do that boosts your energy? For my birthday present this year my family got together and bought me something I have always wanted but not been able to justify – an electric guitar and amp. There were lots of reasons why I should not have got one:

- I can't play.
- I don't have the time.
- We don't have the space.
- The neighbours are already barely talking to us.
- There are other things I could use the money for.
- I've owned an acoustic guitar for over ten years and I hardly ever play that.
- And, I'm too old (from my mother).

In spite of all that I got one. And it was definitely the right thing. A friend of mine found a rock guitar course for us to join and he gave me a lift to the first class. I have since invited others to join the class and afterwards we go for a beer. I had been thinking of inviting two of these friends for a drink for some time but had not got around to it, now the focus and structure of the guitar class has helped to make it happen and Thursday evening is one of the highlights of my week.

The teacher sets us homework each week, which means practice. One day I noticed that when I thought about practising I could almost feel my blood quickening – and you have no idea how rare that is. This, I believe, is excitement, and we all could do with more of it in our lives. That quickening of the blood tells me that not only am I doing the right thing, but I have been putting it off for too long.

WHAT HAVE YOU BEEN PUTTING OFF?

When I ask people, 'what do you *really* want?' they often spend 10 minutes telling me things in a neutral sort of voice. These are things that interest them but the energy isn't there. Then, having got those out of the way, and discovered to their surprise that I'm still listening and interested, they dig a little deeper and often say something like:

- But what I *really* want . . .
- The dream would be . . .
- The ultimate would be . . .
- What I would *really* enjoy is . . .

And their voice is different, their eyes light up, they sit up and the energy is suddenly higher. This is them talking from their heart and for the first time in ages they connect with something half-buried; they feel sufficiently encouraged to share something usually kept hidden, often from themselves. They have postponed it for so long that they have almost forgotten; almost but not quite.

Incidentally, when I told my mother on the phone that my birthday present was an electric guitar, she laughed out loud. I asked why she laughed. She told me I was too old. When I asked why, she told me that I wouldn't be getting the girls chasing me at my age (I had no idea she was so well informed or perceptive). I told her that I hoped she was wrong. She laughed and said she was wrong about everything else, so she was probably wrong about this too.

In identifying what we enjoy, the strength of reaction varies by individual and by activity. The psychologist Mihaly Csikszentmihalyi coined the phrase, 'flow experience', to describe times when people are totally absorbed in what they are doing. Activities are described as either 'high flow' or 'low flow'. Participants doing high flow activities typically report that they:

- Lose all sense of time.
- Are fully engaged in the task.
- Are not self conscious.
- Have a high level of concentration.
- Do it for the pleasure of doing it.

A challenging game of tennis or climbing a mountain can be high flow activities. The focus is entirely on the task they are engaged in and outside distractions do not exist. In a flow experience there is a good match between the ability level and the degree of challenge in the activity – it is neither too easy nor too difficult for them. Athletes talk about being 'in the zone', 'in the groove', or 'unable to put a foot wrong'. I've heard tennis players talk about how the tennis ball just seemed bigger and seemed to move slower that day, as if they had all the time in the world.

At a lower level, we all experience something similar, whether we are dancing, singing, hill walking, gardening, reading a book for pleasure, decorating, listening to music, climbing, playing tennis, speaking in front of a group, doing carpentry, dining with close friends, preparing a report or giving a presentation. Interestingly, watching TV is reported to be a low flow activity.

Doing what you enjoy gives you energy, and should be an important part of anyone's schedule. Yet these activities are often the first to go when things get busy. They seem frivolous, self-indulgent, a waste of time, even selfish, yet nurturing them helps to increase our energy. The paradox is that the time spent on these activities can be self-funding. In other words, the time spent on them is compensated by increased productivity afterwards – because you feel better, your energy is higher, and because you have more energy you get other things done more quickly. One very busy Managing Director I know manages to go the gym or play squash each day. She finds the time spent doing this to be beneficial, because she actually gets more done in the couple of hours left in the afternoon than if she'd spent the whole afternoon working.

Many people have reported that productivity at work goes up after doing activities they enjoy. One person has reported that he is more productive after our coaching sessions. Seeing me takes up half a day, but he finds that he gets more done in the remaining four and a half days than he did previously in the whole week. I can't explain it entirely, but I imagine he has more clarity and focus, that he feels more centred and hears less background noise. I'm not sure he would regard coaching as recreation, but he does see it as an energy booster and it provides an interesting insight into how time can appear somewhat elastic. So if it seems you don't have time to do what would do you good, give it a try and see how you get on.

I used to enjoy doing woodwork, then one day I realised that I enjoyed it more than just about anything else. I used to come home from work, get changed, set up in the garden and get started. Often I did this without even stopping to make a cup of tea, which, for those who know me, is a very significant sign. Yet I was doing it in the garden, dependent on the light and weather. One day, I realised that here was something that I enjoyed enormously and yet I was allowing daylight and weather to determine when and how much of it I could do. So I decided to get a workshop built. We had the space, and it was something I really wanted, but before I could realise my dream there were several steps to be taken:

- I got Rosemary's agreement to investigate it.
- I got rough costs.
- I did a cash flow forecast to demonstrate to Rosemary that we could afford it.

- I identified possible builders.
- I spoke to the planning department.
- I got the neighbours' consent.
- I got firm quotes.
- I picked one builder and gave the go-ahead.
- I supervised the work.
- I acted as liaison when Rosemary asked awkward questions such as, 'Will they use new bricks at the front so it won't match the house? Will the roof be flat or sloping?' (In my haste I hadn't considered either.)
- I got the builders to modify the design (a rather grand term in the circumstances).

It was completed within three months and afterwards I couldn't remember any effort or disruption associated with it. I still use it as a model of what can be achieved if what you want is aligned with something that gives you energy.

> You can have anything you want if you want it desperately enough. You must want it with an exuberance that erupts through the skin and joins the energy that created the world.
>
> *Sheila Graham*

The outrageous is possible if it is what you really want. One of my clients wanted to go skiing more often. I asked how often — he said every week, and I think he meant it. Given he was a family man, I suggested he might want to modify his goal downwards, so he settled for several times a year, starting the next season. I suggested that now he tell his wife what he wanted. He was understandably reluctant, since it seemed a lot to ask of his family. I encouraged him to tell them, but also ask to what he could offer in exchange to make it OK for them. He and his wife agreed that if he took the children by himself to visit their grandparents for weekends that would be OK. He did this, and found the time spent with the children was not only very good for him but also for the grandparents and for his wife. This became a win-win-win situation, and by 24 January he told me he had been skiing four times already that season.

At one time I noticed that, although I was enjoying our weekends a lot, the week seemed to be all about work: doing it, recovering from it or getting ready to do it. So I decided to have a mini-weekend during the week. We allocated Wednesday evenings. I would get home on time, we would have a nice dinner with wine and music, and no TV, and just relax and talk. These dinners were great, and looking forward to them was part of the pleasure – we never felt that far from a weekend. This boosted my energy.

Another of my clients told me that the thing he most wanted to do, which he knew would do him a lot of good, was to play golf, something he had neglected for some time. I asked what was getting in the way. The answer was time. But time has many flavours and this one was tinged with guilt. He said he could go at weekends, but he felt that he would be putting a heavier load on his wife and baby. Alternatively, he could go during the working week, but he would not like to pretend to his wife that he was doing something else. So he would prefer to get her agreement. When I asked why he didn't get it he said that if he asked he expected her to say, 'But what about me? When do I get time to do something I want?'

I pointed out that this response was hypothetical, however likely it seemed. And did he want to let the hypothetical response prevent his checking it out, given how much it seemed to matter? So he asked her, and her reaction was, 'Of course you must play. You work so hard.' Don't let the risk of *possibly* hearing the answer you fear get in the way of asking for something you really want. Children are great models in this regard.

I am reminded of a story about piranha fish in a tank with a glass partition down the middle dividing the tank in half. If you put food in the tank on the other side of the glass partition, then the fish will make a number of attempts to get it but will be prevented by the glass. Eventually they will give up. If you then take the partition away, so they could reach the food, they do not try. They have given up, and in fact will starve to death in the presence of food they could reach. One of the things I take from this story is that sometimes the world moves on, yet our decisions continue to be governed by the way the world used to be and not how it is now. Maybe my client's expectations about how his wife would react to his interest in playing golf would have been true in the past but things had clearly changed and he hadn't checked recently. Where do you, and the people around you, need to update your learning? A clue to this can be found in the language people use. If you hear yourself, or others, saying things such as:

- never
- always
- should
- ought
- can't

then that may be a sign of old learning operating and an indication that there is an opportunity to test the validity of the assumptions underpinning it.

I once overheard some Australian tourists talking about their plans for the day. One of them was inviting the other to join them for a day's sightseeing. The other declined, saying he wanted to do his washing. I was struck by the fact that he did not say: 'I *can't*, I *have to* do the washing', which is what I might have said in his place. In the language he used he put himself in a position of choosing between two things he wanted, which removed some of the resentment I might have felt towards the washing if I were in his position.

OVER TO YOU

1. Make a list below of what you'd really like to do. Take your time over this and let your mind wander. When have you felt really alive? When have you lost track of time? When have you really concentrated? When have you had lots of energy? When have you not been self-conscious? Ask the people around you when you have been like this. What is

it you really want to do? Write it down. Then ask yourself what is it you really, really want to do? Write that down.

My energy boosters

_____

_____

_____

_____

_____

_____

_____

_____

2. Pick one or two from your list and then take a step towards them in the next week. Even if it is a huge thing you want, give yourself permission to want it and to spend some time deciding how to take a step in the direction you want to go. Your aim is to identify a small next step which is 'do-able' and within your control. Consider getting a buddy with a similar interest for support (as I did for my guitar class). I can't overemphasise the importance of doing things with other people – it sustains momentum and helps to dispel the doubts

that surround us, questioning our right to have what we want, our ability to get it, our choice, our competence, and so on. These doubts get stronger when we are isolated, and they get weaker when we join others in endeavours, however modest.

3. Notice the number of times you say any of these words: *should, ought, can't, never, always*. Instead of *should* and *ought* try saying *want*. So if you are used to saying, 'I ought to go now', try saying, 'I want to go now', and notice both how hard it is and what changes occur when you do. Try also changing your language from passive to active. Instead of saying, 'the bin needs emptying', try saying, 'please empty the bin'. On the surface, these may appear to be small changes, but do it a few times and be open to what feels different. Some people report that when they make this change they feel more in control, less stressed, and they stand a little taller.

POSSIBLE BARRIERS TO IMPLEMENTATION

- *I have no time.*
  This really means that you don't think enjoying yourself is important enough to merit finding the time. Start small. Give yourself a treat that you really enjoy, even if it is only for 15 minutes, but make it something that you *really* enjoy, whether it is potting out plants; woodwork; singing along to some music as loudly as you

can; lying down on the floor and listening to your favourite piece of music with the lights off; reading a book with a glass of wine next to the fire; experiencing complete stillness.

- *It would impact the people around me negatively. I would feel guilty.*
  Help them to identify what they would really like to do and offer to support them in exchange. Rosemary and I have supported each other by sharing care of the children so I get to play tennis and she gets to do some gardening.

- *It's selfish.*
  It's part of self-care: and is necessary to recharge your batteries and build a sustainable foundation.

- *I'm too far behind to think about luxuries like this.*
  Even if you only get as far as making plans to do something you really want to do, you may experience a lift in energy. Ever noticed how people's productivity and energy increase just before they go on holiday? It is possible to change gear when you've got something positive to look forward to.

Chapter 8

CHANGE FOCUS

Increase energy by feeling grateful for the abundance already in your life, and stop trying so hard to be consistent.

> At work, you think of the children you have left at home. At home, you think of the work you've left unfinished. Such a struggle is unleashed within yourself. Your heart is rent.
>
> *Golda Meir*

We are pretty problem-focused as a culture – we seem to be able to see what is wrong more readily than what is right. We criticise more readily than we praise. As a result, we all too often live either in the past or in the future, at the cost of living in the moment.

I was once walking with my family round Kew Gardens when I noticed that that particular day there were a large number of people in wheelchairs. It then occurred to me that no one in my family needed a wheelchair – yet. That 'yet' seemed to loom large, and as a consequence I decided to start a gratitude journal – each day I wrote down three things for which I was grateful. It didn't matter what size the good thing was, or if I repeated myself. I wrote what I felt grateful for in that moment. By the end of a month it dawned on me that my life was close to brilliant. People in my workshops often laugh when I say this, as if to say that if it was that good, you must have been a bit dim not to have known already. And they have a point. But the simple fact is that I didn't, and although I imagine that my life is probably not significantly better than the lives of many in my audiences, I suspect that very few of them would consider their lives to be 'close to brilliant'. Nothing external had changed as a result of this exercise, but my appreciation of what I had had changed immensely. We all have access to this perspective; all it takes is a few minutes to see things differently.

Life is good, even when it isn't particularly.

Finding things you are grateful for does not mean that problems disappear. I still had the same problems that I had earlier, and I still needed to do something about them. I still needed to grow the business, finish a myriad of tasks, spend more time with my family and friends, take more exercise. But now my life wasn't just about the problems. It was actually a pretty good life, with some things that I wanted to be different.

At one of my workshops someone complained about the need to get up in the middle of every night to use the bathroom. This elicited the response that she should remember to be grateful that she can just get up and do it by herself. Someone else pointed out this is akin to what her aunt Maud (or some such name) meant when she said 'Count your blessings'. Maybe. All too frequently the message behind that adage is, 'Shut up and stop complaining. Give me a break.' The outcome sought is silence. Whereas the outcome I am suggesting is an increased appreciation of the moment and for the abundance around us.

> There are only two ways to live your life. One is as though nothing is a miracle. The other is as though everything is a miracle.
>
> *Albert Einstein*

Tim Gallwey, the coach and author, asked a great question at a talk I attended. He asked what we were as beings. Someone smarter, and braver, than me suggested that we were beings that had sight. He said yes: we have a visual system that allows us to detect colour, movement and patterns, and to quickly compare the images we see with a bank of others from our past, in order to make meaning out of them and so enable us to take timely action. He asked us to imagine the huge scale of the research and development costs that would be needed to develop and build such a system. The room was silent. We were in awe of something we usually take for granted.

Now imagine housing this system in a unit that is mobile and independent; that can find and prepare its own fuel when it needs it. And imagine making that unit economically viable so it could learn new skills and then sell some of its skills in exchange for the means to buy sustenance and shelter. Then imagine asking this unit how it is, and it replying, 'Mustn't grumble'. If you want to have more energy you need to start being grateful for all the good things in your life. This will help to shift the focus from problems to abundance.

> What a piece of work is man, how noble in reason, how infinite in faculties, in form and moving, how express and admirable in action, how like an angel in apprehension, how like a god.
>
> *William Shakespeare*

STOP TRYING SO HARD TO BE CONSISTENT

There is a myth that you ought to be consistent. What you did before, you must do again, and again, and again. Whoever told us we had to be consistent did us a disservice. The constant effort to be consistent drains our energy and deprives us of some of the opportunities to be spontaneous and more alive. And people with high energy are often spontaneous. In some situations, particularly when dealing with children or managing people, it is clearly important to be consistent, but we may overdo it. In one sense our duty to be consistent could be redefined as being consistent to who we are in the moment, in other words consistently authentic.

> We must be willing to get rid of the life we've
> planned, so as to have the life that is waiting for us.
>
> *Joseph Campbell*

We are not consistent by nature. Have you men ever noticed that shaving at some times of the day is much less comfortable than at others? I once saw an experiment reported on television where a rat was placed in a metal dustbin and a very loud bell was rung outside it. At one time in the day the rat continued to sniff and look around the dustbin apparently unperturbed. At another point in the same day the same bell was rung and the rat died of shock. I don't suppose anyone had told him he was supposed to be consistent.

Carl Rogers, the founder of client-centred psychotherapy, wrote a beautiful classic called *On Becoming A Person*. In the book, he said that one of the major components to becoming fully a person was to be more open to being inconsistent, unpredictable and changeable. As I read that, I find that my shoulders go down slightly and I relax a little more. It is like giving up the struggle to be a certain way and to just be yourself instead. For your interest, some of the other components were:

- Move away from shoulds and oughts.
- Move away from pleasing others.
- Be more open to be all of oneself, no hiding from fears. Be complex.
- Acceptance of others.
- Move towards trust of self.

All of us, at one time or other, have been told, 'That's not like you'. As if to say you've let down the other person by being different from their expectations. The inference is that you need to pull yourself together, rather than they need to accept that you are more complex than they thought. The appropriate response is, 'Perhaps it is.'

Increase your energy by giving yourself permission to be spontaneous and giving up the struggle to be consistent all the time. This does not mean becoming mercurial and unpredictable but it does mean allowing yourself more opportunity to be open to what you really feel.

SURRENDER

Often life does not turn out as we want it to. We have some idea of how we want it to be, and this isn't it. This can lead to frustration and a waste of energy as we struggle to change things. It also reduces our sensitivity to opportunities in the present, since we are more focused on what is lacking. It's like going back to the same resort for a holiday and spending your time thinking about how it compared with the last time – how you remember the beach being cleaner, or the sea bluer – rather than enjoying what is available right now.

But life is a mixture of things both expected and unexpected. Some of the unexpected is welcome, some less so. The choice you have is either to fight the unexpected or to accept it, and with an attitude of curiosity find out how it might be the best thing that could have happened. Losing a job often turns out to be a blessing in disguise for many people, since they frequently find something better or embark on a course of action they would not otherwise have taken.

So when something bad happens, take the opportunity to stop, take stock and then recover from whatever feelings you have about the situation. Accept what has occurred and consider in what ways this might be the best thing that could have happened. At the very minimum there may be something important to be learned from it, and this is the ideal time to learn it. Within the bad news you may see opportunities: the Chinese word for 'crisis' has two characters meaning danger and opportunity.

If life is like riding the rapids down a river, the message here is 'go with the flow'. Use the currents to reach your destination faster, instead of trying to maintain a straight line, which would be more difficult and waste a lot more energy. You can't control or foresee everything, so focus on the present and use it to the fullest.

OVER TO YOU

1. Buy a special book, one that will be a pleasure to write in, and choose one of your favourite pens, or buy one for this exercise. Pick a nice comfortable place and a suitable time of day – early in the day is good, so you can start the day well. Then write down three things you feel grateful for each day and maintain this for a month. Don't wait for a major health scare to appreciate what you have; start now. Oprah Winfrey asked Hillary Clinton how she got through all the difficulties she faced

while her husband was president. Her answer: a gratitude journal.

2. In the evening, write down all the things you have accomplished during the day in a non-judgmental way. Often it is more than we thought. This is a useful technique for reducing the amount of brain space we give to the stuff that is still on the 'Not Done' list, and for appreciating what we have done. I asked one client to do this, who was only aware of what was not done. After maintaining it for a month she was much happier about herself and her business started to take off. It is possible that we will never get to the end of the list, so find a way to enjoy things as they are rather than wait.

POSSIBLE BARRIERS TO IMPLEMENTATION

- *When would I do it in my busy day?*
  At the start of the day, maybe before you get out of bed. Alternatively, after you drop the children at school, or when you first turn on the computer. Find a time that you can make routine so it takes less effort.

- *It won't work, so there's no point trying.*
  How would it need to be different to work for you? Then try it that way.

- *I know I'm well off and I don't need to do this exercise to tell me.*

It might give you more energy to connect with this feeling at a deeper level on a daily basis for thirty days. You can see that you understand something at a deeper level only after you get there. Prior to that you think you understand it. It's a little like listening to my children who, aged nine and eleven, tell me they have done the Victorians, the Vikings and the Romans, and feel they have nothing more to learn about them. My biggest lesson from doing my degree was how little I knew compared to how much there was to know. Prior to that I thought I knew something. Afterwards, I knew that my ignorance was almost unbounded.

- *Maybe* your *life is different to mine — mine stinks right now.*
  I was once sent an e-mail that said, 'If you have food in the refrigerator, clothes on your back, a roof over-head and a place to sleep, then you are richer than 75 per cent of this world.'

  It is almost like we have a 'dissatisfaction gene' that predisposes us to feel crabby. In evolutionary terms, there was probably another branch of humans who spent their time lying on the beach and became someone else's lunch. Our branch survived because we were never content and kept looking over our shoulder. The world has moved on since then, how-ever, and perhaps we can afford to lighten up a bit. We don't need to fear predators to the same extent, we have stout shelters with good locks, and we have the police service, the fire service and insurance to help us with any crises.

- *It's too simplistic.*
  How would you like to complicate it so it works better for you?

- *I don't believe a simple thing like this can make such a difference in my life, so I'm not going to spend a month on it.*
  Why not try it for ten days at a time? Then review and decide whether to continue.

- *It's all a bit new age and touchy feely — I need real solutions to real problems, not mantras or prayers.*
  Assess it on its results.

Chapter 9

SLOW DOWN TO SPEED UP

Slow down to unpick a difficult situation in order to get more done.

FIX THINGS PROPERLY

This one will be a challenge for those of you who think you are too busy. This one can sound like it belongs in the 'nice-to-have-but-no-time' category, and if that is how you feel then it is doubly important that you give it a try. You do not need to commit more than a few minutes a week to experimenting with this one at first and if you like the results you can expand. The concept is this:

Give a problem more time than you think it deserves.

Then get it sorted so it does not come back for years. If a problem merits 2 minutes and is not fixed satisfactorily, then give it 15 and sort it thoroughly. That sense of knowing that it is well sorted increases energy and makes you feel like you are in control and at choice. 'At choice' is a phrase I came across in NLP (Neuro-Linguistic Programming): you can either be 'at choice', where you choose what you want, or you can be 'at effect', where others or circumstances choose for you. When you are 'at choice', you feel proactive, not reactive, and a few experiences of this kind will have you walking taller and getting more done with less effort.

The principle here is to take extra time at the outset in order to save a lot more time later. An analogy is picking up a piece of paper each time it falls off a table − picking it up is the short-term solution. The longer-term solutions are to close the window, use a paperweight or file it away. We often do the equivalent of just picking up the paper and putting it back because we are so busy.

One of the big challenges with this is to resist the pressures to move on to the next thing that is pressing for attention. Most of us have so much to do that even the urgent stuff doesn't get enough attention. The light always feels like it is 'at the end of the tunnel', so the idea that we might find extra time to sort something out thoroughly is a luxury that we can only dream of. I have a lot of sympathy with this point of view. I would suggest, however, that you try it, since the time spent can be 'self-funding' and put you in even better shape to tackle the rest of your 'To Do' list. You feel more powerful when you work in this way. This is not power over others, but power over your circumstances and challenges. People with high energy tend to sort things out quickly.

When it comes to polishing shoes, I often try to rush this and do it with my suit on in less than 1 minute just before I set off. I have also done it the night before and decided to do a really good job and given it my undivided attention for 15 minutes, without the TV. To my surprise, I actually enjoyed it.

You can rush washing your hair, blow drying it in under 15 minutes, or you can spend 25 minutes, using conditioner and mousse, and blow drying it more carefully so it has some shape and enjoy the results all day. You can take the car to the car wash for the minimum wash. Or you can get the most expensive, which sprays the underside, scrubs the wheels and adds wax. Then follow it up with vacuuming the inside, checking the tyre pressure and dusting the dashboard. The latter will give you more energy.

I recently installed some new software from my ISP, but it seemed to have bugs and felt clunky. I called their support line to sort out the first big problem and got it resolved. Then within minutes another problem emerged, this one relatively minor, then another. It was really tempting to give up and live with the minor problems, since there was so much else I wanted to get done. I felt I really did not have the time for this – I had a backlog of several hundred e-mails at the time. Instead, I must have called them six times for different issues over the next two days and got them all sorted as far as possible. It felt great to know that I was not storing up problems that would inconvenience or niggle me in the future, even at the expense of the extra time taken. In the end I decided that the new software was not an improvement and migrated back to the old. And I did it with the confidence that I had given it a good shot, quickly, and got the best help available to try to make it work. The experiment lasted only two days and I moved on without looking back, and without carrying too much of a grudge. I avoided a lasting feeling of anger by channelling my frustration into action and being very clear to myself that they had a limited opportunity to win me over.

Short-term thinking is also one of the common reasons people are sometimes reluctant to delegate. Slowing down is useful here too. People resist delegating by saying:

- They don't have time to spend on briefing.
- It is quicker to do it themselves.
- They can do it better themselves anyway.

All of which is undoubtedly true – for most tasks the person doing the delegating probably will make a better job of it than the person being briefed, especially at first.

Compare this to stopping for petrol but only putting in £1 worth of fuel in order to save time spent standing around on the forecourt. The logic is sound for the short term but makes little sense over the longer term since for a long journey you will have to stop over thirty times more often. Over the longer term, the benefits of delegating are huge:

- We can contribute at a multiple of our individual capacity.
- We have more choices about what to do with our time and can do more of the things we enjoy.
- We grow our people.
- We get to watch them grow – an energy booster for many people.

The challenge in delegating a new task is to remember that you are growing an individual, not just getting the immediate task completed – you are building capability for later use, not for immediate benefit, a bit like planting seed for a later crop.

DEALING WITH STUCKNESS

It can be useful to slow down to deal with being stuck. By 'stuckness' I mean tasks that seem to have been hanging around for a while. They are not necessarily big but they are not being completed, or not quickly. This can include phone calls, writing an important letter or e-mail, or designing something new.

Pay attention to areas where you feel stuck. The temptation is to berate yourself for being stuck, which makes the problem worse. But stuckness is attractive if you can separate the emotion from it. Approach it non-judgmentally, to keep your thinking at a high quality. The attraction lies in the fact that the areas where we are stuck provide us with opportunities for growth. It takes energy to be stuck – energy that is not available for other things.

> All you need is deep within you waiting to unfold and reveal itself. All you have to do is be still and take time to seek for what is within and you will surely find it.
>
> *Eileen Caddy*

As an example, I found myself putting off calling a potential client, having already sent them a proposal. At a rational level, I knew that if I made the call then I would be increasing my chance of getting the business. Why would I *not* want to do it? The resistance, however, was significant, and for over two days I managed to find other things to do rather than make the call and all the while I was quietly criticising myself for not taking action and living with an energy drain. Then I decided to calm down, halt the criticism, and *accept* in an innocent way, without criticism, that I was feeling stuck. Then, in a supportive way, I asked myself what was causing it. Notice that I was not asking myself, 'Why wasn't I getting on with it?', a question that invites a defensive response. Nor was I calling myself names such as: lazy, fool or incompetent. I realised that part of the cause of the stuckness was that I was feeling a bit exposed and somehow 'not ready'. I asked myself what else I would need to feel ready. The answer was that I needed to be clear what further questions to ask them in order to finalise the pricing and also prepare some ballpark prices for the first stage of the project, in case they asked on the call. I worked out these two things, then I phoned them and it felt easy. This whole process took less than an hour, yet I had been putting it off for two days. Having got it out of the way my energy was much higher and the rest of the day went better as a result. By slowing down to unpick the stuckness I was able to speed up. The lessons to be learnt from this are:

1. Notice where you are feeling stuck and accept there is a block.
2. Stop the self-criticism and choose to look at it non-judgmentally.
3. Accept that you are on a journey and this point is where you need to be in order to move on.

4. Accept that there is some important learning in the present situation if you are open to it.
5. Ask what is causing the stuckness.
6. Ask what would it take to be un-stuck.
7. Follow through.

One of the assumptions in this approach is that we are competent but our 'internal critic' can make it difficult to appreciate this at times. The internal critic is a voice that we all carry around in our heads that provides an often-negative commentary on our actions and thoughts. It is the voice that calls us names such as fool, stupid or idiot when we make small mistakes. It is also the voice that makes us doubt our abilities and intentions, sometimes with reason but often without. The internal critic is useful as a signal that there is more work to be done, but often it is overly critical and unfocused. By following this process you take the energy of the internal critic and use it for problem solving. The challenge is to stop feeling battered by the criticism long enough to be able to move into a more rational mode. One way to do this is to use a journal, as described on page 141.

I now have a little Post-It note near my desk that reads:

> When I am stuck, uncertain, unclear or feeling small, look at it non-judgmentally – accept my place on my journey. Stuckness is where my learning happens.

I find this rather reassuring since it has the potential, when I am thinking well and not distracted by doubt, to make stuckness and resistance a powerful ally in my life.

TAKE CONSIDERED RISKS

One way to increase energy and the sense of feeling alive is to slow down, evaluate your situation and then deliberately take some considered risks.

> Most of us tip-toe through life in order to make it safely to death.
>
> *Theodore Roosevelt*

Fear was a big factor in my life. I used to stop myself from attempting things that I wasn't entirely sure about, or I would procrastinate. In my world there seemed to be only two categories of task: things I knew how to do completely and easily; and the rest. The stuff I could do I was intimately familiar with, and the rest was scary. I had this view of the world:

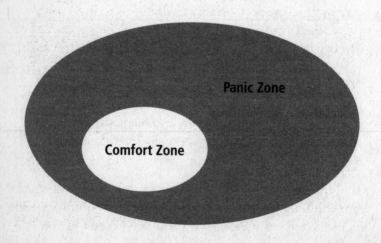

If I didn't know how to do something then I would panic and would delay getting started. I made the assumption that if I didn't have *all* the details sorted out before I started, then I would always fail

As an example, I wasn't sure how to invite a potential client to a meeting in order to catch up on each other's developments, so I delayed making the call – for weeks. Then one day, I was feeling in a particularly good mood and thought I would just do it and assume that it would work out as it unfolded. I did, and it did, and she agreed to meet very readily.

This experience reminded me that there were a few gradations missing in my worldview. A more helpful picture looks like this:

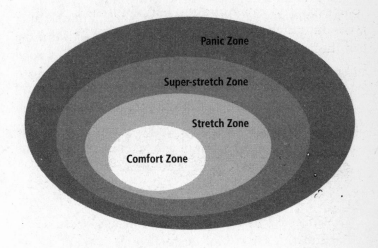

We have the 'comfort zone' of stuff we know we can do easily. One example is driving locally. Outside it is a

'stretch zone': this is where we know part of what to do but it makes us feel a little uncomfortable because it is not entirely within our control or we haven't done exactly this before. An example here is driving an unfamiliar car, in a foreign country where they drive on the wrong side of the road. Beyond the stretch zone lies the 'super-stretch zone'. This is higher risk and getting closer to panic, but there are things here that you know you can do. An example may be the first presentation or speech in your life. You can do it, but boy is the adrenalin flowing. You may know the material but that seems of little comfort when you think about delivering it. Outside that is the 'panic zone' where you may well freeze, run or throw up. In this place you are well and truly out of your depth. An example here is being asked to take over the controls of a helicopter in mid-air without training.

The good news is that risk-taking is like a muscle and, like any muscle, you can build it up. As you take more risks that are considered, not reckless, your comfort zone and your confidence expand, and what used to be a stretch becomes part of your comfort zone. In making the call above I was saying to myself, 'I'm not sure how I'll handle this but I will figure it out as we go along.' At the same time I remembered that fear and excitement are close neighbours and both involve adrenaline.

> . . . and make me climb some mountains, because I need to run the risk of being alive.
>
> *Paul Coelho*

The other bit of good news is that it is in the stretch zones that you grow and learn the most. If you stay in the comfort zone you stagnate. To get the most benefit of the risks you take, it is important to make sure that you stop and give yourself credit for the risks you take. Be sure to congratulate yourself for the risk taken, not the result of the action. For example, take credit for the risk of making the phone call: whether or not you were successful is not relevant at this point.

It is all too common for us to barely pause before we move on to the next task and to miss both the significance and the energy-benefit of what we have accomplished. Build into your day a time to reflect on what has happened and what you accomplished – 5 minutes might be enough to review and give yourself credit; for example, 'Yes, I handled that meeting well considering I've never done anything like that before. Maybe I'm more competent than I think' or 'I knew vaguely what I wanted from that conversation and ended up with an outstanding outcome.'

As you take more risks you also often feel more alive and have more energy. At the low end of the risk scale you could play it ultra-safe: imagine living in a cupboard under the stairs, never going out and having your food brought to you. That would be very safe but a kind of death. At the other extreme, if you did a lot of bungee jumping, parachuting off tall buildings, you would also be risking a more literal death. The ideal is to move the needle a little and feel the frisson you get from doing something which is a risk for you, not necessarily anyone else. Your own feelings are the guide in this, not what anyone else does. If you try to compare yourself to others, there is no way of winning, since there will always be people who are bigger risk-takers and some who are more risk-averse.

DEALING WITH DOUBTS

> Our doubts are traitors, and make us lose the good we oft might win by fearing to attempt.
>
> *William Shakespeare*

Another of the things that drain energy is doubts. In order to increase energy, it is sometimes useful to slow down, to give your doubts your undivided attention and then deal with them fully. This is hard when you are busy, but taking the time to remove unwanted ballast is vital maintenance, necessary if you want to go faster.

Doubts are killers – they cause hesitation and stifle action. They can be severely debilitating, and I should know. I am a world champion at doubt, or I think I am. (See what I mean?) Doubts are little questions or concerns that undermine your confidence and give you pause for thought. Sometimes they are helpful, as in cases of intuition warning you of danger, but at other times they are just an energy drain and a form of self-sabotage.

How do you deal with them? I can suggest three techniques. These are not intended to be a comprehensive answer to doubts, but may be useful to some people, some of the time:

1. *Confronting your doubts*

Doubts seem to have more power when they are vague, quiet and ill-defined, when they give you a sense of being unsettled or unclear. Doubts seem to dislike the light: they are most powerful when they operate at the periphery of our minds, barely in our consciousness. One solution is to bring them into focus, make them centre stage and face them directly, however unpalatable they seem. You can do this by following these three steps:

i. Make a list of all the doubts you have about a certain task. Don't rush, give yourself several minutes to delve and see what comes up. Then write them down, however ridiculous they may sound. Do not censor or edit. The stupid sounding ones have power too, and more so while they remain unvoiced. Make the list as complete as you can before moving on to the next step.

ii. Exaggerate the fear within each doubt, making them worse than they first appeared. Make the fear more extreme, add colour and energy to the doubts to make them more vivid. Make explicit the consequences of each fear.

iii. Reply to each exaggerated fear by asking:

- How true is it?
- What is the evidence?
- Is there an alternative point of view?
- What is to be learned from this?
- What action is appropriate?

To give you an example, these are the doubts I had about a presentation I had agreed to do, that was making me feel nervous.

1. I don't know what I'm going to say at this presentation. I'm going to make a hash of it and look a fool.
2. Some of my clients and potential clients are likely to be there and they will not want to be coached by me. I wish I had agreed to do something safer. This could hurt my business a lot.
3. They wanted something inspiring and I agreed but I think I have overpromised and now won't be able to deliver.
4. This needs to include new material that I don't have. And it will show.

I then exaggerated them and wrote my replies.

1. I don't know what I'm going to say. I'm going to make a hash of it and look a fool. I will freeze and have to walk out. They will all go silent and not talk to me, for ever. I will be embarrassed and will not want to show myself in public again.
   - Well, it is true that I don't know what to say but I haven't started preparing yet. I have found on many occasions recently that when I sit down and start work on something that seems difficult, it turns out to be easier than I thought and I do a good job. Maybe this will be like that.
   - I've also been told on several occasions that I present well. I know lots of stuff that would be of interest to that audience. All I have to do is sit down and prepare, making sure that I give it sufficient time to do a good job. Also it is not just

about the material, it is about how I show up. This takes the heat off the content.

2. Some of my clients and potential clients are likely to be there and they will not want to be coached by me. I wish I had agreed to do something safer. This could hurt my business a lot. I could lose all the clients in the room and a lot of potential clients at the same time. Word might get out and all my clients will want to cancel and no one will ever want to be a client again. I will have to work in a shop.

   • If I stay with letting them see who I am and they do not wish to be clients, then that is good. There is also the very real chance that some will be drawn by what they see and I may attract them as clients instead, which is even better.

3. They wanted something inspiring and I agreed but I think I have overpromised and now won't be able to deliver. They will hate me and laugh behind my back, or even worse, in my face.

   • No, I've given two or three talks to them already. They would not have invited me back if they did not value what I have done in the past. I seem to forget past successes.

4. This needs to include new material that I don't have. And it will show. I should never ever do new material and just stick to what I have done before.

   • But what is now old material was new once. I took a risk then and it paid off. Maybe this will be the same. Imagine if I could develop this new stuff into a new programme which becomes an additional service and income stream. This is exciting. I've been looking at the downside and forgotten that the reason I'm doing this is to take risks, to develop new services that I can test in relative safety and attract new clients. I'm over-focused on the negatives.

With that, I felt much better about the presentation. It will still be a risk but the risk seems smaller and worthwhile since I have connected more strongly with the positive.

2. Identify the key limiting assumption

The second way to deal with doubt is taken from Nancy Kline's fabulous book *Time to Think*. This also involves three steps:

i. Firstly, when you feel a doubt about a situation, ask yourself: 'What am I assuming that is getting in the way of feeling positive?' The answers will be limiting assumptions and they are usually fears about the outcome. If there is more than one, pick the one that feels like it has the most weight.
ii. Secondly, create the 'Positive Opposite' of that assumption. This is an opposite that is desirable and stated in the present tense.
iii. Thirdly, craft the 'Positive Opposite' into an 'Incisive Question', in order to ask yourself what you would do differently if you knew this opposite to be true.

An example from my journal will illustrate this. I was about to go to a lunch meeting to meet two people in a firm of accountants. One of them was a partner and he had previously seen a presentation I had done on coaching and invited me in to talk further.

1. I have low energy about this meeting today. What am I assuming about the meeting with this firm?
   - That they won't buy anyway and it doesn't matter what I say.
2. What is the 'Positive Opposite' of this?
   - They will buy if it is the best thing for both sides.
3. What would I do differently if I knew that they will buy if it is the best thing for both sides?
   - I'd relax and engage. Treat the potential contract as an issue we share and we jointly have to decide whether to go forward and how. Not take it personally. Focus on what they are looking for and how to help them and then later decide whether coaching is the appropriate solution to their needs.

This changed my outlook hugely and took just 5 minutes. The meeting went very well, and even though they did not go ahead with the coaching, I enjoyed the meeting.

3. Journal

As will be ascertained from the above, another tool for reducing doubts and increasing energy is to keep a journal. Many people recommend this, and so do I, as it is a place to think through concerns, feelings and thoughts you have about your life and forthcoming events.

The most common formula is to buy a special notebook, find a quiet place and write daily for half an hour. I write mine on my PC, to improve my typing speed, anywhere from one to eight times a week. Often I use it to think through something about which my feelings seem to be inappropriate, for example when I am overly scared, overly relaxed, tired, lacking energy. At other times I use it simply to pay attention to myself – what is going on in my body and where, what am I feeling and thinking. It is one way of clearing my mind and centring myself so I feel less distracted, more ready for the day ahead. I recommend it highly. I also use it to give myself credit for achievements and risks taken. Other points to bear in mind when keeping a journal are:

- Writing in the morning is better than later on as you will find you talk more about feelings and less about events.
- If you are not sure where to start, try asking some of the following: What are my feelings right now? What do I notice in my body? What thoughts or incidents keep coming back to me? How do I feel about yesterday?
- Don't worry if you miss a day or three, just resume when you can.
- Make an agreement with your partner that the book is private and off-limits.
- Do not explain in the journal – no one else will read it. You don't have to read it either. You can, but it is not necessary to feel the benefit.

OVER TO YOU

1. Notice if a problem keeps recurring but you don't feel that the time taken to sort it out would

be worthwhile. Slow down, set a budget for how much time you will spend on it and make sure it is more than you think it merits. Then give it your full attention to get it sorted and feel the difference.

2. Make a list of all the things about which you are currently feeling unsure or have doubts about. Pick the one that you have the most energy for, or the highest interest in. Then set aside some time to deal with that item, and make sure that you aren't interrupted. Pick the technique that most appeals to you and give it a try. You may not need to go through the whole of the technique – you can stop when you feel your energy has increased and you are ready to take action. Pay special attention to the internal signals that tell you that your energy is high.

POSSIBLE BARRIERS TO IMPLEMENTATION

- *What kind of risks should I take?*
  Pick small ones to begin with. You will know they are risks because they make you feel slightly uncomfortable when you think about doing them. Examples might be paying someone a compliment or asking a small favour of someone. Make sure that you build in time to appreciate yourself for the risk taken. Otherwise you will lose a big part of the cumulative benefit.

- *I have too many doubts to use these techniques – I'd never get anything done.*
  Start chipping away by taking one situation at a time. You don't have to tackle them all in one go. Maybe do one a day or one a week.

- *I'm not convinced about the journal thing.*
  The best way to find out is to do it for a month and review the results.

Chapter 10

ON HAPPINESS

Three ways to be happier and have more energy.

Happiness is hard to hold on to.

> Twenty-three hundred years ago Aristotle concluded that, more than anything else, men and women seek happiness . . . . Much has changed since Aristotle's time . . . And yet on this most important issue very little has changed in the intervening centuries. We do not understand what happiness is any better than Aristotle did and as for how to attain that blessed condition, one could argue that we have made no progress at all.
>
> *Mihaly Csikszentmihalyi*

There is a strong link between happiness and energy — when you feel happier you usually have more energy, and vice versa. I am no expert, but I have picked up a few clues about happiness. They don't cover all situations or all people, but they may have relevance for some people, some of the time.

HAPPINESS IS A CHOICE, NOT A CONSEQUENCE

This is the first clue. This means it is available now and is within your grasp. It is a shift in attitude that is at once easy and, at the same time, hard. And for those of you who feel that there *is* light at the end of the tunnel, but it seems to be taking a lot longer than expected to reach it: maybe the light will never get any closer and you might as well start enjoying what you have.

Obstacles

For a long time it seemed to me
that real life was about to begin,
but there was always some obstacle in the way.
Something had to be got through first,
some unfinished business;
time still to be served,
a debt to be paid.
Then life would begin.
At last it dawned on me
that these obstacles were my life.

Bette Howland

My wife and I were driving to a fortieth birthday party. We had had a normal busy day, had got changed in a hurry, then briefed the babysitter, given the children a goodnight kiss, probably had to prise one of them off us, and dashed out. I was driving slowly over the speed bumps so my wife could put on her lipstick in the car. After a pause, I turned to her and told her that I had just realised that I was not looking forward to the party. This is the awareness stage – not to be undervalued since all deliberate change starts here. She said that she wasn't either. We were too tired, and too rushed, and could really have done with a quiet night in with a glass of wine, in front of the TV.

However, a bit of me was also telling myself that a party is usually seen as a nice thing, that probably people had gone to considerable trouble to organise this one. So what on earth were we doing setting off feeling so low? What kind of life was this that we let ourselves feel so stale and jaded about going to a knees-up where we would meet up with a lot of our friends?

Another pause. Then I had a radical thought. 'Shall we just decide to enjoy the party?' We both paused while we considered this. Mostly I used to go to parties and, based on what happened, decided whether or not I had had a good time. Usually afterwards.

A second question followed, 'Can it be *that* easy?' That was a bit scary, to have that much influence over our experience. Well, we both decided to enjoy the party. And one of the consequences was that I dumped what had happened earlier in the day at the door and entered the party determined to be as fully present as possible. The result? We both had a great time. During the evening I reminded myself more than once that I had decided to enjoy the evening. My energy was high, I felt playful and everyone seemed interesting and attractive. It was light years away from how we had felt at the start of the evening.

It *was* that easy. It took a few minutes to notice what we felt, to reflect on it, and then to choose a better alternative. In NLP terms we had an 'outcome orientation'. In everyday English, we had made a decision that predisposed us to have a good time.

This incident reminds me of the truism: 'I'll believe it when I see it'. In this instance, I adhered to the reverse, 'I'll see it when I believe it', in other words the belief that I would enjoy myself came first, and thus made the outcome more likely to happen.

> The one fact that I would cry from every housetop is this: the Good Life is waiting for us – here and now.
>
> *B. F. Skinner*

To make this work in your life you need to find time to reflect, to notice what is going on within and to make decisions based on that. For this you require quiet, since it is not possible to hear what your inner self is saying if you are always surrounded by noise. In the above example, we did not have the radio on, nor were we trying to fit in a discussion about Christmas presents or anything else. We had a quiet few minutes to settle and, although I was driving, I was still able to become more aware of my feelings. I now recommend that people do not always turn on the radio when driving, so that they are able to listen to what is going on inside. It is surprising how involving this can be, so involving, in fact, that the radio is hardly missed.

Many events are outside of our control, yet how we respond to them is, to a large extent, within our control. Some people who get cancer say it was the best thing that ever happened to them. It shifted their perspective and it became much easier to see what was important to them. They were grateful that the disease gave them time to put things in order.

When something bad happens, such as rejection, once the initial hurt is over, we have a choice. We can choose whether to continue with the pain and resentment, or we can start looking for what was good about it. One positive aspect may be that the rejection did not happen any later, which would have wasted more time.

I was discussing the subject of happiness with a colleague when he asked me, 'Are you happy?' This stopped my pontificating in a heartbeat. I had to think, and was surprised I did not seem to have a ready answer. My reply was, 'I am when I remember.' And that's one of the keys – we need help to remember to choose to be happy.

True happiness comes not from the absence
  of problems.
True, enduring happiness comes in spite of
  the problems.
Happiness is not a reaction, it is a choice.
  Let it be yours.

Ralph Marston

PROGRESS TOWARDS GOALS

The second clue is this:

We feel happier when we have clear goals and a sense of making progress towards them.

This is one of the key findings from several studies into happiness. It may seem deceptively simple, but don't be fooled. There are two parts to it and both have challenges.

The first part is to set goals that are achievable, relevant and motivating. What we're not concerned about is the nature of the achievement – it is more about feeling happier, so the actual goal is less important than the principle of having a goal – almost any goal.

I want to emphasise three points about this. Firstly, goals can be small. There's a huge benefit to be derived from completing small goals that are 'quick wins' in terms of feeling happier, and it pays to write them down first. Small goals can be anything from making a phone call, doing the shopping list, to running an errand.

Secondly, it is sometimes hard to think of goals, since, for many people, the very word carries a certain amount of unwanted baggage. If this is true for you, then try asking yourself:

- What would need to have happened for me to feel satisfied with my day/week/month?
- What's not working well?
- What changes do I want to make around here?
- What needs to be different?

Take any one of these approaches, make a list, then rate your list out of ten for satisfaction, i.e. 'How satisfied will I be out of ten if I do all this?' If you come up with a rating of ten then you are ready to start. If the rating is less than ten then ask yourself what else would be needed to get it to a ten. Then repeat the exercise until you get to a ten (or nine, if you don't ever think you'll get to ten).

Thirdly, don't criticise yourself about your choice of goal. Your internal critic may tell you that the goal is not big enough, that it is unimportant or too easy – 'Anyone could do that! Call that a goal? Is that the best you can do? Are you going to base your happiness on that?' Just tell the critic that you're doing an experiment, you'll review it later, and thank it for its input.

> It is good to have an end to journey towards; but it is the journey that matters in the end.
>
> *Ursula LeGuin*

This idea of goals and progress is reinforced by something my doctor once said. I had asked him if I might be depressed – I'd read one of the leaflets in the waiting room and thought I recognised some of the symptoms. (I've since stopped reading them.) He told me that I was definitely not depressed. Then I said I had a problem with low self-esteem at times. His reply was: 'We feel good when we are fit and dynamic.'

That made me stop and think. I thought I knew what 'fit' meant – regular exercise, and that sort of thing. But 'dynamic'? I decided it must mean becoming the master of your own destiny. By this I mean setting some goals and making progress towards them. In doing this you become more proactive and less reactive. You start to exercise your right to choose. You decide what you want to do and then start doing it. It was a recipe for life. I loved the simplicity of it, and it became my mantra.

At the time, I was working in marketing, and I decided to put my new philosophy into practice. So I set aside some time to think, and imagined that I was a year in the future doing a review of the year that had just passed. I asked myself what I would need to get done in order to feel satisfied with the past twelve months. The answer came quickly: get six to eight initiatives off the ground. That seemed very clear and energising. If I could point to half a dozen projects that I had initiated, some of which had made a profit, then I would feel very pleased with myself, and also have something for my CV, whether I was looking for a move internally or externally. My new found enthusiasm and energy carried me over the immediate obstacles of deciding which projects to tackle, and finding the time to do them.

I solved the first problem by asking my staff to tell me which projects they would like to implement and to provide me with analyses of the costs and benefits. I used these to prioritise. Then I had to deal with my boss. He had a tendency to treat everything as a priority, so I decided that I would need to take the initiative. I sat him down and took him through the eight projects I was keen on and, with the financial justifications, explained why they should be priorities for the business. He accepted them all as priorities. Then I took him through the nearly 200 other items on my department's list. He confirmed that they all belonged on my list. As I was leaving, I told him that I would make sure the eight big projects happened, but that there might be some casualties among the others. He was silent, so I continued walking.

That was it! I had got his consent, or as close to it as I was going to get. I then made these projects my first priority and implemented all of them over the next year. And felt great doing it. I had lots of energy and really felt clear about where I was going and how to get there. In the end most of the projects, though not all, made a profit. And what about all the stuff that didn't get done? I didn't hear much about it, so it probably wasn't all that important.

The lesson to be learnt from this experience is to create for yourself a satisfying year. Start with the end in mind and consider what needs to have happened for you to feel good about the twelve months just passed. With that kind of clarity you increase energy enormously. If you'd like to read more about this, see Jinny Ditzler's excellent book *Your Best Year Yet*.

Six things

Here is an energy-giving idea on a more modest scale. Pick six things you intend to do the next day. They can be small. This is one of my typical lists:

1. Send agenda in advance for meeting next day.
2. Confirm meeting later that day with one client.

3. Chase my wine order.
4. De-fragment the hard disk on the computer.
5. Bring two boxes of books in from the car.
6. Put the books on the shelves.

I completed this list by 10.10am and had high energy for the rest of the day! The items were not all work-related, nor were they all urgent, and one, the wine, was downright trivial, but my mind was sending me a message that I had had no response from the shop. Part of me was saying, 'Never mind, it's expensive, so it's probably just as well', but the voice wouldn't go away. Having responded I felt great. And although my priority is work, my brain and the resulting energy level do not seem to know that.

So is this just a trick of putting up easy tasks in order to feel more energy? Yes – it's a quick win with no side effects, and it's cheap. The tasks don't have to be easy, but it helps. Remember the benefit you want from this exercise is more energy, not mountains moved. Although, once you have more energy, it will become easier to deal with the mountains.

A few points to bear in mind:

- Write the six items down so you can see them.
- Write the list the day before so when you get up in the morning you have a clear sense of direction and momentum.
- Put a line through them as you do them.
- Make them easy – do not set yourself up for failure.

One hundred wants
This is another energy-giving idea, which is a development of this theme. Write down a list of 100 things you want before you die. This can be a challenge for some at first, but it gets easier with time. You can include big things and small things. Then decide which you would like to get done within the next three years. One woman I know drank a glass of bourbon and smoked a cigar, neither of which she actually enjoyed but she wanted to do them. Another of my clients made a list and within six months had completed a third of them.

ARE MOST PEOPLE HAPPY?

The third clue concerns a misperception many of us have: that other people are happy. They look happy, or at least happier than us. This is based on the fact that we know intimately what is going on inside of us, but know only part of what is going on in the lives of others, and, in comparison, they look pretty together. This assessment is false and drains energy. The truth is that most people are not that happy – they are waiting to get through something first. The very phrase 'The pursuit of happiness' in the American Declaration of Independence implies that happiness is elusive, effortful and carries no guarantee of success.

If you are struggling with problems, it is a real downer to believe that most other people have got it more sorted. This means that as well as all the difficulties you already face, you can now add being inferior. It is hard not to compare ourselves to others, it's probably part of being human. Other people may manage to put on a great act of being pretty together, but when we scratch below the surface, we can get a glimpse of the cracks and challenges. This is enormously reassuring. It tells us that in this regard we are pretty much like everyone else, that there is nothing much wrong with us, and we start to go a little easier on ourselves.

We have more in common in our problems than in our accomplishments. The world is full of quiet heroes: people getting on with their lives and doing well in spite of huge challenges and difficult circumstances that they don't talk about. It's a shame they don't talk about them, because the experience of sharing can be validating for all of us, and could be the start of people helping each other.

So if you are feeling like you are less happy than others, ask around. Just ask people: 'Do you think most people are happy?' This is a less intrusive question than starting with: 'Are you happy?' You'll find that most of us are in the same boat. That the majority have lots of things that are right with their lives, but also things that make them dissatisfied. On balance you've probably got it about as right as most others.

Chapter 11

CHILDREN AS
ENERGY DRAINS

*Some ideas to use to reduce the energy-draining
moments that involve children.*

Unfortunately, as joyful as they can be, children can also
be a huge energy drain, requiring an enormous amount
of repetition, cajoling and negotiation to get even the sim-
plest things done. Why can't they just do what you tell
them? First time? Then there are all the regular trouble
spots: mornings, meal times, bath times, bedtime, tidying
up time, car journeys, etc. Were we like this?

For me, having children was a much better, and much
worse, experience than I had imagined – the highs were
much higher and the lows much lower. The highs are difficult to match in any other way – that depth of love, the
freshness with which they see ordinary things, the unmod-
erated enthusiasm for simple pleasures, the energy and
immediacy of their interests, the deep healing quality of
their hugs, and the animal warmth and 'rightness' of their
cuddles, gratefully received any time they are on offer.

And it brought out a tenderness in me that was long buried, like watching my heart go out raw into the world.

The challenge is to shift the balance so that you have more of the good times and less of those that drain energy. How do you contain the routine maintenance and training activities so that you can spend more time doing, and be in a fit state to enjoy, the soul-nourishing stuff? I take mine to school three days a week, and there have been some mornings, after dropping them off, that I have needed to lie down for 10 minutes to recover. 'Yes, I do want you to take your coat. I know it's sunny now, but take it anyway just in case. It's not stupid. Yes, it does look unlikely that it will rain, but it might.'

However, things have changed a lot recently, and I was amazed to find myself one morning reading a book, almost serenely, while they were getting ready for school. I suddenly realised what I was doing and it struck me how much things had altered. How was this magical transformation brought about? The following is part of my personal experience from various parenting courses that I have been on and from books and tapes that I have consumed. The most useful course by far was run by an organisation I can heartily recommend: The New Learning Centre in London (see the Resources section for contact information). These are some of the things we do that work in our household. You may need to amend them for your circumstances. At the time of writing, my children are aged nine and eleven, and they are pretty normal – the usual mixture of wonder and woe.

DESCRIPTIVE PRAISE

Children spend so much time doing things that we don't want them to do, or at the wrong time, that we can end up sounding critical and negative: 'Stop that. Hurry up. Fold your napkin. Careful you don't spill your drink' etc. This makes us, and them, feel bad.

A powerful alternative is to praise the behaviour you want to see more of. The key is to be specific, so they know exactly what they did right, which makes it harder for them to argue with and easier for them to do on another occasion. And praise also the absence of the negative behaviour; so if they are not squabbling, not playing with their food, not eating with their mouth open, then tell them. The reward for them is your pleasure and the positive attention you lavish on them. We use this a lot, when we remember. One of the challenges is to be sufficiently present and aware so that we have enough brain space available to notice and praise. The temptation, when they are not misbehaving, is to move on and modify some other aspect of their behaviour, or to just get on with your life. Some examples from our home may help:

- Thank you. I heard every word you said. You didn't mumble at all and I feel less tense because I don't have to strain to hear you. It makes such a difference!
- Thank you for not tilting your chair back.
- You've put your shoes away without me reminding you.
- You put your coat away as soon as I asked, even though I know you wanted to go on the computer.

- Well done, you got completely dressed and I only had to ask you once.
- Thank you for waiting while I finished my sentence, even though I know you were dying to speak.
- Well done, I can see that you wrote really carefully and neatly. I can read every word and all the letters are on the line.
- You're being very patient.
- You are behaving at the table so much better. Do you remember I used to sit here and feel a knot in my chest at meal times? I haven't felt that in a long time. You are interrupting, shouting and grabbing less. I guess you're growing up.

What do you praise? Start by choosing which aspects of their behaviour you want to change. Then look for opportunities to praise even the smallest step in the right direction. There are so many things that children can be praised for, that we have been able to praise ours for ten separate things before breakfast.

ONE-TO-ONE TIME

This is a technique that demonstrates to children that they are important and helps to build their confidence and self-esteem. It is also a way of creating a special time which, when it works well, increases energy.

One-to-one time is a predictable period of time set aside to spend just with your child, doing something together. During this time you are implicitly telling your child that they are a priority in your life and that you are actively choosing to spend time with them. The time is predictable so that the child knows it is coming and can bask in the anticipation rather than have it just sprung on them as the mood takes you.

What do you do in this time? In our home, we negotiate: I ask them what they would like to do and I tell them things I would like to do. Then we spend half the time on one person's preference and half on the other. Recently, I took my son on a trip to the dump to drop off garden waste for my chosen activity and, for his, we wrestled. It worked well for both of us.

How long do you need? We aim to do anything from 15 minutes to an hour several times a week with each parent. Occasionally, it might be something special, such as taking one of them to watch the tennis at Wimbledon. The dream is one hour each day with each parent.

The challenge with this is finding the time and making it regular. However, it is important and the effect is lasting. I deal with coaching clients who, although they are highly successful adults, still feel at some level the lack of time spent with their fathers. Steven Biddulph, who writes on child development, has said that if you are working fifty-five or more hours a week the development of children into balanced adults is at risk.

SOLUTION TALK

This is a startlingly simple and powerful tool, which continues to make life easier and can also, I'm told, be enjoyable, assuming you're not too tired before you start.

Rosemary and I have tended to start these talks at 10pm, which is a time we are both likely to be in, but this is too late to enjoy them. So we are looking to find a better time.

We aim to spend 15 minutes a day where we briefly name a problem area and then brainstorm solutions and agree a plan to implement. The goal is to agree the problem area within a minute or two. This is not a time to whinge and moan. Then the rest of the time is spent on what we can do to make things work better.

An example might be: how do we get our son to put his napkin in his lap and sit straight in his chair at meal times? It is so boring and annoying to be reminding him each time and it just does not work. He obviously couldn't give a monkey's, and that somehow makes it even more annoying.

By focusing on a problem daily, and coming up with a solution, we get a terrific sense of progress, which helps to increase energy. We also get an enhanced sense of our own competence, so our self-esteem goes up.

By the way, the answer to the above problem is to hand him his plate of food *after* he is sitting straight and has put his napkin in his lap. Works every time. The challenge for us is to remember to do this each time and to not be so preoccupied with dishing up and getting to our food while it is still hot that we forget.

DEALING WITH BOREDOM

'I'm bored.'

Oh, how the heart sinks and the energy flags at this announcement. One technique is to focus not on solutions and activities, but on the child and their mood. So I will ask them lots of questions that narrow down their interests, and then give them choices. I find it does not work to give them suggestions, as they are not receptive, my efforts are unappreciated and I get fed up. It's important to give them your whole attention while you do this, and not attempt to do the cooking or read e-mails at the same time. This is an example of a conversation with my daughter:

'I'm bored.'

'Good, so you're bored. Do you want help from me to decide what to do?' (Show no emotion, even if inside you are feeling 'Oh no, not again! How many toys does one child need?')

'Yes.'

'Do you want to do something inside or outside?'

She turns to the window, pauses and says, 'Inside.'

'Upstairs or downstairs?'

Pause. 'Downstairs.'

'Active or not active?'

Pause. 'Not active.'

'At the table or somewhere else?' By now the idea has come into my head that painting might be fun for her, so I offer choices that head in that direction.

Pause. 'At the table.'

'Writing or drawing?'

'OK, I know what I want to do, bye.' And off she goes, in a very different mood. And I am dismissed.

I can't remember whether she went off to paint or draw or to play with Lego. I don't really care at that point. My job was to help her recover her resourcefulness and connect with herself. The moment she goes off with a sense of purpose my job is done.

The pauses are significant since they allow her to reconnect with herself and discover for herself what she wants. It's almost as if by saying she is bored she is saying she is feeling unsettled and unfocused and can't think straight. My job is to help her thinking improve, not to find her something to do to solve being bored. This cannot be rushed – part of the solution is the quality of your attention and patience.

ENCOURAGING SELF-RELIANCE

As parents, one of our main roles is to be a teacher. Within that, one of our most important jobs is to foster self-reliance in our children, so that they are better prepared to be independent as adults. One way we do this in our home is to ensure that their pocket money is *earned*, not given. It is earned by carrying out certain tasks around the house. Below is the kind of chart we use to help us do this.

Term time

		Sun	Mon	Tues	Wed	Thu	Fri	Sat
Morning	Get dressed	☐	☐	☐	☐	☐	☐	☐
	Make bed, sort clothes, floor clear	☐	☐	☐	☐	☐	☐	☐
	Breakfast	☐	☐	☐	☐	☐	☐	☐
	Face, teeth, hands, hair	☐	☐	☐	☐	☐	☐	☐
	Prepare lunch box		☐	☐	☐	☐	☐	
	Empty bins	☐						
Take	Indoor PE kit				☐			
	Outdoor PE kit/shoes						☐	

		Sun	Mon	Tues	Wed	Thu	Fri	Sat
	Check plant	☐			☐			
	Call Grandma	☐						
Meals	Clear table	☐	☐	☐	☐	☐	☐	☐
Home	Shoes away	☐	☐	☐	☐	☐	☐	☐
	Coat away	☐	☐	☐	☐	☐	☐	☐
	Lunch box cleaned		☐	☐	☐	☐	☐	
	Hang up backpack		☐	☐	☐	☐	☐	
	Everything done today?							

If they get everything done they earn their pocket money for the day. For each item they miss, they lose a portion. You will need to design one for your children that addresses the friction points in your home.

What difference has it made? The chart is on the wall at child height and they can look for themselves to see what they need to do, so we are not repeating ourselves. We used to be almost nagging: 'Have you done your teeth? Got your homework? Got your PE kit?' Not any more. The incentive of earning pocket money has taken care of the motivation issue and the visible checklist has dealt with most of the need for reminders. Initially if they were not sure what to do, we simply asked, 'How can you find out?', and after a moment's thought they remembered to look at the checklist. After a while they stopped asking.

Getting my children to talk to my mother on the phone each week was a challenge. It was somewhat easier when they were younger, but more recently they seem to have other things they would rather do. By putting it on the list we now get much more compliance and it is barely an energy drain to get it done. Before we put it on the list, whenever we did manage to get them to the phone, they would say 'Hello. Goodbye', and hand the phone back to me. Now that we have specified that we need at least 2 minutes of conversation, and in a pleasant tone, they are much more willing to do it and my mother is delighted.

This way of working teaches the child self-reliance, which is better for us as parents, and them as future adults. It also means that we are in a better mood, so if the children do get ready early it is possible for us to play together before school, and we actually feel more like it. In the summer we have even gone to the tennis club behind our house and played tennis for 15 minutes before school. On other occasions we have played a board game or done some painting or woodwork together.

It may seem that this method is totally reliant on money as a reward – it is not. We use the opportunity of checking the checklist with them to praise them for completing tasks. And the praise matters to them. While it is a shame that money has any place as a reward, it is a fact that, at the moment, this is what seems to work in our home.

Our checklist, above, may seem a little daunting at first. We started small and built up. One of my clients saw this on our wall and implemented something similar in his home, but had just seven items, including: Be nice to your sister. Behaviour improved significantly and instantly. Modify the concept to suit your home.

We allowed my son to earn the micro scooter he desperately wanted by earning points for doing extra homework, and by doing it with good grace. A few days after he got his scooter he said that he felt good about it because he had earned it, whereas other children had got theirs by nagging. I feel good that my children are beginning to learn that they can earn the things they want by their own efforts.

GETTING MORE COOPERATION

If people, and this includes children, are not cooperating it usually means there is a block in either will or skill. If the problem is skill then the solution is either more training or more development, i.e. they may not be mature enough to tie their shoelaces or drive a car. If the problem is will then it may need some ingenuity to find a motivator that works. Descriptive praise (see earlier) is one such motivator and there may be others that work in your home.

One of the things my children are very keen on is *The Simpsons*, and they like to watch it every day. So we use their enthusiasm for this to help us in something we wanted, which was more cooperation around the house – more help with chores and the following of instructions first time. This was particularly important when we wanted them to get out of bed in the morning – both children climb into our bed in the morning for a family cuddle and we bought a six-foot-wide bed to make the most of this opportunity while it lasts. However, getting them out of our bed and dressed is still a challenge. Another challenge was leaving friends' houses and leaving the After School Club. Departures could take anything up to 20 minutes.

The deal we came up was this. In order to earn *The Simpsons*, there had to be five incidents of cooperation during the day. Each incident gives us a chance to shower them with praise for behaviour we would like to see repeated. The result is that we have much better co-operation and they have never missed the chance to watch *The Simpsons* (partly, it has to be said, because we make it easy for them to earn it).

RULES OF THE HOUSE

Children have a great skill in testing us – it is partly their job, to test limits. They are quick to spot inconsistencies, unfairness and the hesitancy in your 'No'. They force you to think about values, principles and morals. And it can be hard work, since so many situations have precedents and may have repercussions later.

Another device we use in our home is to have a clear set of rules for the house. You need to design a set that is appropriate for your home, but here is a sample from those that we use. It is important to write them down and make them visible since it is so easy to forget what the rule may be in any given situation. One of the benefits of rules it that they clarify expectations and help to make life easier.

Rules
  1. Cover mouth and turn away when coughing or sneezing.
  2. Squabbling happens in your bedroom or at the far end of the garden.
  3. Go to bed on time.

---

4. Be in the same room as the person you are speaking to.
5. Be honest.
6. Laugh with people not at them (no 'Ha Ha!').
7. Sweets at home on Fridays only.
8. Ask permission where appropriate with other people's stuff.
9. Make amends if you damage someone's stuff.
10. No name calling.

Every so often, we review the rules with the children and let them have their input. This is a chance, usually at the weekly family meeting, to check clarity and fairness and to get their commitment. The rules also give us an opportunity to praise the children for good behaviour. They provide us with a prompt to look at what they are doing and see what we can praise them for. So, for instance, even if they are eating with their fingers, we can praise them for having all four chair legs on the floor.

LUNCHBOX CHECKLIST

This is a different use of a checklist and you may need to develop your own version to make your life easier and the children more self-reliant.

Making their lunchbox started when they were seven. It can be hard for children, as there is a lot to remember, so I sat down with them and together we came up with a checklist to make it easier. The list is below.

How to make a lunchbox

1. Put lunchbox on counter.
2. Put in fresh fruit.
3. Get crisps or peanuts.
4. Get water container, fill.
5. Get treat (apricots, cereal bar).
6. Put in ice pack.
7. Get from fridge and put on counter:
   • lettuce
   • roll
   • cucumber
   • salami
   • mayonnaise
8. Get equipment:
   • chopping board
   • sharp knife
   • spreading knife
   • box and lid
   • rubber band
9. Build the sandwich and put in box.
10. Zip up and put by front door.
11. Put leftovers back in fridge.
12. Put dirty equipment by sink.

It took a while for this to settle. I soon noticed that they were not using the handwritten list I had put on the wall and, when I asked why, they told me they couldn't read my writing. I had always thought I had pretty good handwriting, but in this they were clearly the judges, and as I was not getting the result I wanted, I knew I had to change. So I typed the list and put it up again. Still they weren't using it, and I decided that the writing was probably too small, so I made it bigger. Now one of them uses it regularly and the other does not seem to need it. It took maybe three months to get to this point. It sometimes takes time and experimentation to find a solution that works.

Why all the checklists? Some of you may be wondering if we even have a checklist for the bedroom: place tissues within reach, clothes off, get into bed, prepare for impact of cold feet. (We don't.) Checklists save the time and energy wasted thinking about the same uninteresting things many times over. They save our children asking us what needs to be done, and all of us thinking too much about routine tasks.

Chapter 12

ASK FOR HELP

Involve others in your projects if you want to feel increased energy.

This can sound odd.

How does asking for help increase my energy? Surely it would reduce it by making me feel helpless and hopeless? Others will think less of me. What if I don't need help? I've never asked anyone for help and never will.

If you don't need help, then maybe you really don't need help, but sometimes we can overlook our own needs because we are so used to wanting not to be a burden. One way to check if help would be useful is to ask yourself:

- Where in my life am I dissatisfied with the progress I'm making?
- Where am I a bit blocked?
- Which problems do I wish would just disappear?
- My life would be a lot easier if . . . (complete the sentence).

- What needs to be different for my life to be perfect?

Use these questions to help you identify where help may be useful. There is no assumption here that you are weak or damaged, rather that you want to make faster progress. Working with others can speed things up and the process of asking increases energy.

There seem to be a number of reasons why asking for help increases energy:

- You connect more with your network of contacts.
- You give others a chance to give, and giving raises energy.
- Others are flattered you asked, and you have paid them a compliment in asking.
- You build community and get to feel more connected with the world.
- You tell people in a natural way what is happening in your life.
- It is a basis for chatting, and many of us don't do enough of that.
- You take action.
- You share some of your vulnerability, which can be engaging

It is hard to ask for help, especially for men, but also for anyone who learned somewhere along the way that they had to 'be strong'. I attended a workshop where the facilitator started by talking about his lifetime achievements and career highs, some of which were notable (several marathons, mountain climbing, business successes). Then, by contrast, he surprised me by listing his lifetime lows, such as the death of a close relative, divorce, bankruptcy. I was impressed by the highs (thinking that's probably a better list than I could come up with), but I didn't actually start to warm to him until he talked about his lows. That's when he became more human and we had more common ground. Peter Ustinov once said, 'We admire people for their achievements but we love them for their failings.'

When I was given the contract for this book to sign by my literary agent I felt confused. Being new to this sort of thing I had no idea whether what I was being asked to sign was favourable, standard or outrageous, and I wasn't sure how to sort it out. I read it with a rising sense of dread, then read it again with a sense of despair as the legal language and implications were not becoming any clearer, despite my persistence. Then it occurred to me that I was trying to do this all by myself, and I didn't have to any more. I started asking around and e-mailing people, using the opportunity to let them know that I had had an offer from a publisher – something that part of me really wanted them to know, but which I had found very difficult to drop into conversation. The problems I was having gave me a legitimate excuse to share my good news. I contacted a lawyer friend who did not have expertise in this area but he asked a colleague who did and who owed him some favours. A few days later I received a four-page fax from an industry expert which was very reassuring. I was knocked out by the generosity. As side benefits, I added a lovely sounding lady to my network and made more public my commitment to get this book finished.

I once met a fellow coach at a networking meeting and felt that we had a rapport. I called him up a couple of weeks later and asked him if he would be interested in doing some co-coaching to help keep each other focused on business development. I was afraid of appearing needy, of looking like I lacked friends and feared being rejected. He, however, agreed readily and said he was pleased I'd called. We've been talking weekly for four years now and he is one of a group of people I look to for support. If there is something you want, try asking for it. People are surprisingly responsive if someone else makes the first move.

> Ask, and it shall be given to you; seek, and ye shall find; knock, and it shall be opened unto you.
>
> *Matthew* 7:7

I needed some new glasses and decided to get help in choosing them as I wanted to eliminate the feelings of doubt I had about my previous pair. I hired a superb image consultant called Esra Parr, who is based in London and is part of a national network (see Resources for contact details), to first do a consultation and then accompany my wife and me to an optician. It felt great, and different, arriving with 'my team'. After an hour we picked the glasses. Has anyone made a comment on them, favourable or otherwise? No, and that is fine. I am confident that they don't do anything horrible to my face and are the best that were available in that shop. What this process has done is eliminated a potential energy drain: it has allowed me to stop wondering, or doubting, whether these glasses suit me. In this instance, asking for help was a form of doubt-reduction.

OVER TO YOU

1. Set aside 15 minutes to make a list of all the areas in your life where:

   - You are feeling a bit stuck.
   - You are not making the kind of progress you would like.
   - You feel blocked.
   - You don't know how to proceed.
   - You feel uncertain.

2. Pick one or two areas for which you have some energy.
3. Identify someone who would be willing to help. It's not necessary for them to help you directly – so long as the will is there it doesn't matter if the skill isn't.
4. Call them up and tell them that you're looking for someone who might be able to help with a couple of situations. Describe the situations and ask who comes to mind. As you speak, a different part of your own brain will be engaged and the right person may pop into your head. Start optimistically – assume you will get it

> sorted somehow and they, or someone they
> know, may be able to speed up the process.
> 5. Contact this other person. Do this a few times
> and see how you get on.

POSSIBLE BARRIERS TO IMPLEMENTATION

- *I don't think I need any help, thanks. I'm doing fine.*
  We can all make faster progress with a little of the
  right kind of help. This obstacle may be fear – see
  below.

- *I wouldn't know who to ask.*
  If you're not used to asking for help it can feel difficult at first. This may be fear talking. You may feel
  safer initially asking someone with whom you already
  have a good relationship, or perhaps e-mail him or
  her.

- *The people I know don't like helping others.*
  Then start with others – don't set yourself up for
  rejection.

- *I don't know what kind of help I need – I'm stuck. I
  wouldn't know what to ask for.*
  If you want to try out this technique, then talk it
  over with someone you trust. Sometimes we get so
  stuck that we can't see what kind of help might be
  useful, but, to someone else who is less involved, it
  may be blindingly obvious.

- *The world is a competitive place – you just don't do that sort of thing.*

  That is purely an opinion, which means it can be changed. It is an opinion that does not serve you well: it does a little, in a protective sense, but it carries a price. The price is that the barrier is indiscriminate. As well as protecting us from the bad stuff, it keeps out the good. For instance, by keeping our distance from strangers we are less likely to get involved with unsavoury characters, but we are also going to make fewer friends.

Unfortunately, there is no way of being that does not carry *some* price or risk. It seems a shame, but it's also potentially liberating, since if all beliefs carry a price then we may as well give up the pursuit of the one that is perfect or completely safe. Let's concentrate instead on playing with as many as we can until we find one that serves us better than the one we used before.

The phrase 'playing with' can cause difficulties. It is a little like being told to relax. I hate being told to relax or lighten up because it is often advice that I can't use; I need to hear the 'how'. I was once rehearsing part of a presentation for a sales conference when the producer and my managing director both told me that I needed to project more. I knew that already, but presumably they thought it was new information, or at least I hope they did. What I really needed to know was *how* to project more. There was a gap between wanting it and knowing how to achieve it. At the time I wasn't able to articulate my need and they didn't ask – a simple 'Do you want to know some techniques for projecting?' would have helped.

But perhaps they didn't know how either. I wish it was easier to ask for help.

There are lots of blocks to asking for help. In my primary school, at the end of the day, we used to put our chairs on the desks (presumably to make life easier for the cleaners) and then say the Lord's Prayer. The chairs had a gap between the back and the seat. On one particular day, it seemed like a grand idea to see if I could get my head through the gap. By moving slowly and turning my head to the side I made it and was very pleased. At the end, the teacher was furious and told me to come up to the front and say the prayer aloud, by myself. Silence. She asked again. More silence. Long pause, everyone wanted to go home and I was holding them up. I could feel the animosity building up behind me. Then, bless her, she asked if I knew the words. I shook my head. She offered to say it out loud and gave me the chance to repeat it after her. This I did and we all went home. She was wise and must have known that my behaviour was not rebellion but an inability to comply or ask for help. For some reason I did not feel it was acceptable to tell her that I did not know the words after years of apparently reciting them. I'm still pretty pleased with getting my head through though.

Although I am suggesting that you experiment with asking for help, I find that when people say, 'lighten up' or 'play with an idea' it makes me constrict and tightens my energy. What works better for me, and may work better for you too, is to think of it as an attempt to:

Reduce the weight of the consequences.

How does one do this? One obvious way is to create more opportunities so, if the current one fails, you have more to turn to. I sometimes get anxious before making sales calls to potential clients. One way of deflecting this anxiety is to increase the number of people I call. If I only have a small number, I worry that I might blow them all and be left with nothing. Then my mind starts to move quickly: I face the prospect of the collapse of my business; the shame of another career failure; the loss of my livelihood, my mother saying, 'What kind of job was it anyway for a grown man with a family?'; losing my home and family, living on the streets, etc. If I have hundreds of prospects left, however, I am less concerned and may even be grateful if some of them say no. This is an abundance of opportunity. (For more on this, see Chapter 8).

Another example is the single person looking for a partner. Often they get pretty nervous about the first meeting with a potential partner. Underlying this anxiety is an assumption that they will not have many more such opportunities and that if this doesn't work out, it means they will remain loveless the rest of their lives. If, instead of that thought, they could replace it with an assumption that they will be seeing a thousand potential partners, then the consequence of any one not working would be considerably reduced. As a by-product they will be more relaxed and the meeting will probably be more successful than it otherwise would.

The world is competitive at times and cooperative at others. The good news is that you can choose which belief to keep front of mind as you engage in any activity. It makes sense to choose the one that is most enabling.

Someone defusing a bomb could either choose to keep in mind that the bomb might go off or that they have defused many others. Both beliefs are true but one is going to help with the job in hand and the other will interfere. If you choose to believe that the world is mostly a friendly place, then it will be easier to ask for help and feel the benefit of increased energy.

Chapter 13

SURROUND YOURSELF
WITH PEOPLE WHO BOOST
YOUR ENERGY

*Spend more time with people who boost your energy
and less with those who drain your energy.*

One of the major influences on energy is the people in
your life. You know how you can really look forward to
seeing some people and others make you sort of wilt?
Some people drain you and others lift you. Some can see
the negative in things whereas others can see what is
positive.

When you are around people who lift you, you
somehow feel cleverer, wittier, more confident and attractive, and the world is your friend. They bring out your
best and the effect can last for hours or even days afterwards. You hold them in your heart and thoughts even
when you are apart and you feel they do the same.

People who drain you have the opposite effect. When
you are around them you feel smaller, uncertain and pulled

down. These are the people you dread having to see and they affect you even when they are not around. Just *thinking* about seeing them or talking to them drains your energy. They are a drag to be around and you imagine their lives can't be any fun. These are the sort of people who, when you ask how they are, may say:

- 'Not *too* bad' (meaning pretty bad nevertheless).
- 'Mustn't grumble' or 'Can't complain' (much as I'd like to, given half a chance).
- 'Not dead yet' (might as well be).
- 'Hangin' in there' (not sure why).

> I have worked with a lot of people who have life-threatening illnesses, and when they faced death, they all discovered the same thing: time isn't money, it's everything. Spend it on who and what you love.
>
> *Bernie Siegel*

I want you to make two lists: people who lift you and people who drain you. Include work, personal contacts and people you come across casually. Also include those you meet fleetingly, such as the librarian, other parents outside the school gates, neighbours, people at the tennis club – they all have an impact. This is not just about life-long relationships, these are people who occupy some space in your world and are a part of your environment. I am embarrassed to admit that I seem to have taken a vague but strong dislike to one man who works at our local library. I don't know why, but I am clear that he has a draining effect on my energy and my day is definitely brighter if I don't have to deal with him. I now choose to renew my books over the phone in order to reduce contact with him.

After you have compiled the lists you may be surprised or embarrassed by the findings. That is OK at this stage; just tell the truth as you see it. Perhaps one list is much longer than the other? How many of your family are drains? What about your partner? Some people may appear on both lists – look for the patterns to identify specifically when the same person is a drain or a lift: what are they doing or talking about, who else is present and might it be related to location?

The next step is to decide who you want to spend time with. Are you spending as much time as you want with people who lift you and as little time as you want with the other group? If you are, congratulations. If you are not, then plan to spend more time with those who lift you and plan it in as a priority. For example, do you want one nurturing contact each month, week or day? My recommendation is that you start to shift the balance or make an adjustment so you have more exposure to people who lift you.

I told a former school friend that it was ridiculous we were not seeing each other more often given we were now living thirty miles apart. We were only meeting once a year, in a good year. Previously, we lived hundreds of miles apart and, for three years, thousands of miles apart. So, at my instigation, we got out our diaries and planned a year of meetings at six-week intervals, alternating venues and whether it was a family occasion (lunch) or for adults (dinner). And there was something nice about knowing we had a year of getting together already planned. That was treating it like a priority. Then other arrangements were made to fit around these arrangements. And if an opportunity arose that we wanted to take up, and which conflicted with one of our scheduled meeting days, then we would renegotiate the date for our get-together and move up or down by a week.

Some people object: 'I don't have time, what with two jobs, children, parents, the shopping, business travel, keeping a house.' I know it is hard, but it may be possible to sort something out that is time-efficient. I arranged with two people that we could call each other up during the working day to have a chat. We specifically agreed that we would do no admin on the call, such as arranging a time to meet. The point of the call was to make contact. We agreed that the call would last no more than 3 minutes, if that was appropriate. It worked well. Once I got through to one person's secretary who told me that he was in a meeting and asked if I wanted to leave a message. I said I did and it was, 'Hello'. She told me that that had made her day. So not getting through touched three people that day.

Often these people were in meetings and we found ourselves swapping voicemail messages over a few days before we connected. One nice thing about this was that during those days we knew that we were in each other's thoughts and we knew that the calls came from the heart.

WHAT DO YOU DO WITH THE PEOPLE WHO DRAIN YOUR ENERGY?

Before you consider changing the relationship, it is important to use some introspection and ask yourself what factors have caused the relationship to feel like a drain. Are you perhaps a drain for them? Sometimes priorities change and the changes can reduce the 'fit' between people. An all-consuming job, new children or a new partner can all affect relationships and may just be temporary. On the other hand, it may be that the other person is simply different in a way you don't like – they may have a tendency to disagree with everything you say, or enjoy debate or be very confident or bouncy all the time. This does not make them wrong, just a poor fit at the moment, and you need to take care of your energy level as an act of self preservation. If the effect on you is significant then it may be worth looking at the following options.

Having decided that some people are a drain, and that you want to do something to lessen their impact on you, how do you go about it? There are three choices and I suggest you start at the top first.

1. Help them to be less of a drain.
2. Accept them as they are.
3. Drop them.

With option one, you become proactive by changing your attitude and behaviour first. When you make a change, the other person is often forced to do something different and that can create a more positive relationship. The change starts with you, not them, and it requires a change in behaviour, not just a complaint.

When I told one wag about these options, he asked me, 'So what do you do with your mother-in-law? You can't drop them.' True, and maybe this is one relationship that has to fall into the 'Accept' category. First, however, you need to do all you can to minimise the impact by negotiation, for example, agreeing with your partner that if you spend X amount of time in her company you've earned the right to do Y (but make this something you want to do which does not look too obviously like avoidance).

Alternatively, you could help them be less of a drain by taking the approach adopted by one memorable client. He told me that his mother-in-law was coming down to stay that weekend and he was not looking forward to it because the relationship was, at best, superficial and, at worst, tense. I asked what kind of relationship he wanted, and he said he wanted to talk about things that mattered more. I asked what he could do, what behavioural changes he could make, to move the relationship in the direction he wanted. He suggested he could start by making her feel welcome when she arrived. I asked how he would do that and he suggested getting in her favourite brand of sherry and telling her he had done so. I asked what else he might do that would help move the relationship in the direction he wanted. He decided that he would wait till he and she were alone in the house and the others were having a tour of the garden. Then he would casually pick up a picture of his wife as a young girl from the mantelpiece and ask if she remembered when it was taken, and use that as a starting point to talk more about his wife's younger years, which interested him and he knew would interest her.

By the end of the call I could feel that his energy was higher, and he was actually looking forward to her visit, so that he could put this plan into operation. My energy was also higher, and I could hardly wait to hear the results.

When we spoke the next week he told me the weekend had been a great success and that his in-laws had extended their visit (a first) and stayed on for an extra two days (a result he was pleased with, although in my workshops this gets some laughter about whether it should be called a success). They had gone to the races together and he had taught her how to place bets and he said that she was walking to and from the betting office like an excited little girl.

As well as using strategies to promote a different kind of relationship it is sometimes possible to train people. My mother is a bit of a drain, which sounds kind of unfortunate, to say the least. However, I decided to do something about it. Firstly, I told her that I sometimes left our phone calls feeling a bit down, since much of what I was hearing was complaints about her acquaintances, the home help, the central heating engineer, etc. And by telling her, I gave her information she did not have – that her behaviour has an effect, that it is not always positive, and it may not be what she intended, if she intended anything.

If I had left it there I think I would have been in trouble. However, I had a suggestion for her, one that was probably going to be a bit of a stretch but worth a try. I asked her to start the phone calls with good news. She replied that she didn't have any good news and, from her point of view, that is believable. But I don't give up easily. So I once asked:

'What did you have for lunch?'

'Dahl and rice'. (She sounded puzzled – why would I want to know?).

'Was it nice?' I asked. (Hoping this might work. Not sure where to go if it doesn't.)

'Yes'. (Still puzzled.)

'Well that's good news!'

Then she started to laugh. And after that the whole conversation felt lighter. And since then, bless her, she will sometimes remember this and start the call by saying, 'I have some good news, you want good news, here is some good news: I've found someone to cut the grass and he will only charge £5.' And it makes such a difference to me. She is less of a drain and is more aware of the effect she can have on me. She also comes to the calls with more energy, which is infectious.

For my part, I have involved her in my work. She has no idea what I do and each time I explain her eyes start to glaze over. My mother has a charmingly simple view of work: there are three jobs in her world – lawyers, doctors and everything else. She has never really understood what I do since our worlds are so far apart. I wanted to feel closer to her, but this lack of understanding was a bit of a barrier. So the way I did it was to get her support, to ask her for something that she would understand and want to give. Whenever I am going to an important meeting or on a business trip I will phone her beforehand or from the airport, and let her know that I am going to an important meeting and ask her to wish me luck and send me her blessing. She is delighted to be able to offer this and I feel more connection with her and a little less alone in those key meetings. It works for both of us. And it may be the first thing in my adult life that I have asked of her.

She recently asked me if I had found someone else to call to wish me luck, since I had not done it for a few weeks. I reassured her that I had not, but had simply forgotten. I have since resumed.

With some people, just giving them some *gentle* feedback on how you are affected by them will give them pause for thought, and may be enough to bring about a change. This may be information that is new to them, that no one has bothered or been brave enough to give them before.

Others, however, will continue to be oblivious and may require more of a nudge. Try making an enquiry to elicit suggestions from them first – if the suggestion comes from them they are more likely to carry it through. For example, try saying, 'I sometimes leave our phone calls feeling a little low. Were you aware of that? How do you feel hearing that? How do you feel after our calls? I *do* want to talk to you and I'm wondering what we might do differently so that I feel that way less often.'

If they don't come up with anything useable, you might want to consider making a request. If, for example, a person is a persistent complainer, you could ask them to restrict their moaning to a certain number of minutes, so that after that you could talk about other things, or hear some good news or hear about what is going well in their life. Ask them, 'How do you feel about that idea? Would you be willing to try it?'

Option two is to accept them as they are. If none of the above has worked and you fear that they are not going to change in spite of your best efforts, then you still have some choices before you consider cutting them off:

- Reduce the frequency of contact.
- Change the location.
- See them in the company of others, hence diluting the effect.

- Find a pastime that interests you both and will create some diversion, such as the cinema or a concert.
- Live with it. You can regard the energy-draining effect they have on you as just part of the price of being alive – the almost inevitable grit in the sandwich when you have a picnic on the beach.

Option three, drop them, usually gets the loudest protests in my workshops. It sounds harsh and some people have difficulty with it. 'How could you?' 'How cruel!' 'Isn't that when people need you the most?' 'That's what friends are for.' There is usually a strong unspoken sense of duty in these protests, a strong 'should'. We need to reduce the number of 'shoulds' in our life and increase the 'wants'.

It is possible that by dropping people who drain your energy you are doing them a favour, since you are creating space in their lives to replace you with someone more rewarding. Conversely, you may be slowing them down from a better life by being 'nice' to them. Dropping them may hurt in the short term, but long term there is a real chance that both of you will be better off, as you may have been a drain on them too. By dropping them you are sending a message that something they are doing is a turn-off, and the sooner they get the message the sooner they can review what they are doing and make an adjustment. That adjustment may lead to them creating much more significant relationships than the one you have ended.

This is analogous to some advice given by Thomas Leonard, coach, author and founder of Coach U. He recommended that one should not coach alcoholics. This was because, although in the short term, coaching could make their life better, it would delay the freefall necessary for the alcoholic to reach rock bottom, get the message and then start on the road to real recovery. So coaching in this scenario would be a palliative that slows down the eventual cure.

Here is a tricky question. Can you dump an old friend? I tried to upgrade the quality of relationship I had with one old friend. We had known each other for over fifteen years. I had lived with him for a month while I was between homes, and some weeks we had socialised several times. He was a successful businessman, and I had seen his name mentioned more than once in the *Sunday Times* as a leader in his field. He had once said to me that I was his best friend in London and intimated that I was not living up to that role since I was not often available. So I arranged to see him more.

One day, as I walked away from a restaurant where we had had lunch, I noticed that I was more aware of the amount of time the lunch had taken out of my day, than I was of the pleasure I had derived from spending time with him. I realised that this person had become a 'should' for me, and that I was seeing him partly out of a sense of duty.

So I made a plan. I decided that next time I would ask him an important (for me) question to try to build more intimacy. I had tried to do this in the past in half-hearted ways, but with no success, and I still wanted to alter the relationship so that it was more rewarding for me. The question I came up with was, 'What are your hopes or fears for the next year or so?' I planned to ask it at a moment that seemed most likely to get a response, when we were both comfortable and relaxed. His answer mattered a lot, since, depending on his reply, I was either going to drop him or have a very different relationship – I couldn't continue as it was. The idea of a different relationship was exciting. As far as I was concerned this was one final attempt to nudge him into a fuller relationship. His reply was disappointing: 'Don't have any really.' That did it for me. I've not seen him since, and that was over five years ago. We are still in touch, I invited him to a party and we exchange Christmas cards, at which level the relationship is not a drain. I may contact him again at some later point to see how things have developed.

To soften the blow of dropping someone, given that your friendship may be more important to the other person than it is to you, it may be worth seeing if you can introduce them to others who share similar interests. You can use your network to help connect them to people they may have more in common with.

THE 5-MINUTE MIND DUMP

One idea for getting more energy from your main relationship came from Peter Senge, the management guru. The idea is that both of you – ideally at the start of the evening – sit down somewhere where you can give each other your full attention for 10 minutes, with each of you getting 5 minutes in turn to talk. One of you starts and just talks about how the day was, what the journey home was like or whatever else is at the forefront of your mind. The job of the listener is to listen. The speaker specifies what kind of listening they want, for example:

- sympathy ('poor you')
- attentive silence
- summarising
- questioning for clarity
- appreciation ('well done you!')
- and last, and definitely least, advice

The listener has to fulfil their brief for the full 5 minutes and be comfortable with silence if necessary. Silence does not mean lack of activity. Allow the other person to enjoy silence with your attention, if they want to. Imagine how refreshing that could be. The important thing to avoid is giving advice when it is not sought. This has a way of irritating people and breaking rapport. The speaker is free to change their mind, however, about the kind of listening they want during their period, for example, after a few minutes, they may then want advice, but it is entirely up to them to say so. No interruptions should be made unless invited.

By giving full attention means that nothing else should be done at the same time – no opening of the post or looking through the TV guide or cooking. The time is to be treated like a high priority. You must spend the time looking kindly at the other person and making every effort to look encouraging and interested, even if you don't feel it.

RAISE ENERGY THROUGH BRIEF CONTACTS

> Call it a clan, call it a network, call it a tribe, call it a family. Whatever you call it, whoever you are, you need one.
>
> *Jane Howard*

We humans love contact or interaction with others. This does not mean just physical contact, but also making a connection, or having one's existence acknowledged with a look, a smile or a 'Hi'. The need for contact is so strong that we will sometimes risk negative consequences in order to get it, for example when children are naughty or squabble in order to get attention.

Deprivation of contact is damaging. Laurens van der Post wrote several books about the ways of the Bushman people in Africa. One of their most extreme forms of punishment was for the community to literally turn their backs on an individual, refusing to acknowledge their existence. And many of us know how uncomfortable it can be to be 'sent to Coventry', even in jest.

The converse is also true – you can raise energy by having positive interaction with someone else. Apart from the need for contact you can raise energy by having a series of positive contacts in your day. I happened to be in the front garden and I got two smiles from the woman who delivers the free local paper, in spite of herself: one when I said a loud 'good morning' (she must be used to thinking of herself as invisible) and another when I said 'thank you' as she was leaving.

Start a conversation with the person at the Sainsbury's checkout. One thing is for sure, and that is that you are going to have to spend some time standing at the checkout. You might as well make the most of it. Not everyone who works at the checkout is a joy to talk to. So I start with a hello and smile and, if it seems right, I might then go on to make some comment that is true for me, for example, 'It seems quiet today, is everyone watching the rugby?' 'Had a long day?' Or, more risky, 'Did I see you looking away as I approached, hoping I would go to some other till (said with a laugh)'? Some respond and some retreat. Those who respond lift my day. And I'm OK with those who don't – they probably have other things on their mind and I don't take it personally.

Take advantage of the opportunities the day presents to make contact with people. Say 'Morning' to that other cyclist at 6.30am in Richmond Park. Say a friendly 'Hello' to more of the other parents at the school gates.

I am reminded of what one country dweller said – he could always tell the city folk. They would look at you all the way as you crossed a field then turn away just as you got close. Try saying hello and notice the effect on you. It may be subtle, but it is an important contributor to your energy level.

The written word also works beautifully as a form of contact. I once sent a note to thank a secretary for the way she and her colleague took care of me when I went to her company to do a presentation. I sent it to her Managing Director. One possibly surprising thing is how good it felt to send it. You get energy by giving. I keep a fountain pen and a nice notepad for such notes, which I use in preference to e-mails.

I also invited a mother and her daughter I knew slightly from the After School Club to my home for a cup of tea. As a consequence, my daughter and hers have become good friends. With these and other steps I am expanding my community. It can be tempting to say I am too busy, but this stuff recharges the battery, gives you more energy, and it is in these moments that life is lived.

On the tube I noticed a woman sitting opposite me trying to see the title of the book I was reading. It might have been a self-development book such as *Make Your Life Stupendous In 7 Minutes* or something similar. I might even have felt mildly embarrassed, imagining that someone who saw me reading it would think: 'What a loser! Not only must his life be so crap that he is trying to change it, but he must be really desperate if he thinks he is going to find the answer in a book.' Then I remembered that, as unique as I am, there are many ways in which I am similar to some others and wanting a better life is probably one of them. So I took a risk. I held up the book so she could see it clearly and smiled. She smiled back and that was it. I carried on reading and she carried on looking around. A nice moment and a bit of contact. It made the world a more friendly place to be. How many of these opportunities are available to you?

OVER TO YOU

1. Make two lists of people – those who lift you and those who drain you, include work and personal contacts. Also include more peripheral

contacts, such as the librarian, other parents outside the school gates, neighbours, people at the football club. Become protective about who you let into your life and how much you will allow them to affect you. Find a way to spend more time with the first group. Build a community of people who lift you.

People who lift me	People who drain me
PETER MOST OF THE TIME	PETER WHEN HE TALKS ABOUT JOANNE
MICK	JOANNE
STEVE	RECEPTIONIST AT XYZ
MAN WHO WALKS DOG	PLUMBER
TENNIS COACH	NEWSAGENT
ARCHITECT	TICKET PERSON AT UNDERGROUND
STUDENTS	EVENING CLASS TEACHER
GARAGE MECHANIC	LAWYER
SOME SPECIFIED COLLEAGUES	OTHERS
SPOUSE (WHEN?)	SPOUSE (WHEN?)
SOME FRIENDS	OTHER FRIENDS

A community is where you are seen as a gift.
Julio Olalla

Couldn't we all do with more of that? Peter Senge echoes this point. He advocates finding a partner at work to help create a learning organisation:

> . . . *your prospective partner should be a 'nourishing person' for you: someone whose face lights up when you walk into the room and who has few, if any, plans for your improvement. Partners may have a vision of your potential, but they thoroughly accept you as you are now. As you sort through the close relationships in your life, you may discover that only one or two people meet these criteria — and your significant other or spouse may not be one of them!*

2. Looking at the people in the first group, pick some you would like to spend more time with. Then arrange to see them or call them to tell them you really enjoy their company and would like to have more contact with them. If they respond as you hope, you can then have a conversation about how that might work given your schedules. Set up some arrangement that works for both of you.

One of my clients wrote on his preparatory material, prior to the start of coaching, that he had never had a mentor and felt the lack. I asked him to pick who he would like. He picked someone he had only met once, but knew by reputation and was very impressed by. We talked through some of the doubts he had about approaching this person and, the next day, he invited him to lunch. They talked through what he had in mind and the other person accepted the role of mentor. It can be that simple.

3. With each person in the *second* group, decide what you want to do: help them to be less of a drain; accept them; or drop them. Then set aside some time to plan by yourself or talk through with a coach, or a significant other, what approach to take to make things work better for you.

These changes are possible and often much easier than you think. A lot of problems we put up with can be solved by simple focus: I don't want this; I want it to be more like this. What can I do to get it there? One of the reasons problems persist is that we don't give them the attention they merit, we move too quickly on to the next thing. (For more on this, see Chapter 9).

4. Take one opportunity a day to make extra contact where you might not have done so before. And notice what you feel. Practise on supermarket staff, on staff at the Post Office, or anywhere where you are waiting with other people: at the bus stop, outside the cinema, at the station.

5. If you experience good service from someone, take the time to tell them or their supervisor. Send a hand-written note – some people recommend sending five appreciative notes a day, even if only to a friend to say 'Just thinking of you today . . .'

6. Start building your network and sense of community by reaching out to people. A lot of people are just waiting to be asked. You will feel more energy when you feel connected to a large community. Take opportunities to make and build your community.

POSSIBLE BARRIERS TO IMPLEMENTATION

- *Isn't dropping people all a bit brutal?*
  I recommend that you do not drop people without trying several different approaches to elevate the quality of the relationship first or to dilute the effect on you. Ultimately, this is about self-care. I also wouldn't recommend dropping people who are going through a temporary problem, only those who have always been a drain for you, even if you weren't always aware of it.

- *Isn't this all a bit selfish?*
  Yes and no. It is about self-care: the healthy end of selfish. You need to take care of yourself so that giving to others doesn't eat you up, resulting in burnout. If

you don't take self-care seriously, you risk becoming a bigger drain than the people you were helping.

One of the things you need to do is to learn not to compromise too early. Compromise is, of course, part of growing up and is healthy for society. Young children do not compromise and it can be hugely wearing on others. As we grow up, we learn that we can't have everything we want, as soon as we think of it, and we learn to postpone gratification, an essential emotional skill that can predict later success in life, according to Daniel Goleman, author of *Emotional Intelligence*. We learn to fit our wants and needs in with those of others. So, for instance, it is helpful that children learn to have a 'precautionary pee' before going on a car journey. They may not need to or want to right at that moment (they'd rather carry on playing), but it may save everyone time and trouble later. This is a helpful example of compromise.

The danger is that we sometimes overdo it, and start putting what we imagine to be the needs of others before our own. We might think that we are supporting someone by listening to them ad nauseum, and that, at some point, they will be ready to do something about their situation. So we sit there, swallow our frustration and listen, because we want to be loyal. However, some people seem to be perpetual complainers and have no intention of changing anything – they are more attached to complaining than to making their situation better. Jack Canfield, who co-wrote the *Chicken Soup for the Soul* series of books, calls these people 'Energy Vampires'. With these people, rather than just listening, it can be helpful to

204 High Energy Habits

give them a nudge to action. If they really have no intention of making changes, it starts to become questionable what you get out of the relationship.

- *Aren't you meant to help people who are drains?*
  If their drain phase is temporary, then it makes sense to hang in there and support them over a difficult time, in the same way that you would like to be able to count on the support of your friends in trying circumstances. If, on the other hand, they have always been a drain, then other action may be called for. If you are genuinely happy to just listen, then it may be appropriate to continue to support them. But for most of us, we do this with a grudge, not with pleasure. So it is an energy drain. You may be able to help them more by getting out of their lives and letting them build relationships with people who do not see them as drains, who appreciate them more.

- *Doesn't all this take a lot of time?*
  Making the list takes only a few minutes, and picking up the phone to call one of the people who lift you will also only take a few minutes. Once you've done these two things you are on your way. It can feel refreshing and powerful to call someone up and tell him or her that you really like their company and would like to have more contact with them. Do not let the busy-ness of your daily life deprive you of the nutrition you need. At the end of your life, which are you more likely to remember – the tasks or the relationships?

  You need to realise that these nurturing people are as vital to your well being as food. If you are so busy in your hamster wheel that you don't have time available to spend with people who are good for you, then what is the main point of living? Is it just about survival? If so, life must seem more like a punishment than a reward and opportunity.

Remember, also, that short encounters can be immensely rewarding. A friendly word with someone in a queue, with someone's assistant or with a receptionist can change your whole mood in a moment. Be open to these brief gifts: they take very little effort and time. If someone provides a service you appreciate then take a moment to ask him or her their name (this is a compliment in itself if asked in an appropriate tone) and tell them exactly what they did that you liked. Leave a trail of appreciation wherever you go. Most of us do not get enough appreciation, so, when it is given, it has a disproportionately beneficial effect both on the recipient and on us, the giver.

- *I'd be too embarrassed to tell someone I want to spend more time with them.*
  Look upon it as taking a considered risk, the by-product of which will be an expanded comfort zone.
  – For more on this, see Chapter 9.

- *My partner may want something different.*
  Check it out. It is surprising how often people make assumptions about their partner's view and find it erroneous, so start by checking it out. If it turns out they do want something different to you, then talk it over and negotiate a solution that works for both of you – find some give and take.

- *I'm too busy to talk to store staff.*
  You're going to spend time waiting in the supermarket or in queues anyway. You might as well make
  the most of it.

  - *I don't get enough appreciation myself. I can't give it to others.*
  By giving you do not deplete yourself – the act of
  giving is also beneficial for the giver. It's a shame
  there isn't more appreciation around, but you have
  the chance to do something about it.

> It is one of the most beautiful compensations of life
> that no man can sincerely try to help another
> without helping himself.
>
> *Ralph Waldo Emerson*

Chapter 14

IMPLEMENT THE IDEAS YOU HAVE ENERGY FOR

Here is a checklist of some of the ideas in the book to help you get started. If they are something for which you have a lot of enthusiasm, tick the box in the first column, if they interest you, tick the box in the second column. Those you tick in the first column are the ones to start with.

	Lots of enthusiasm for	Interested
Fix those little things that you've been ignoring	☐	☐
Clear the clutter	☐	☐
Build in reserves of time	☐	☐
Create thinking time each week	☐	☐
Spend more time with people who lift you	☐	☐
Five-minute mind dump	☐	☐
Create a checklist of new daily habits	☐	☐
Pay more attention to the 'little voice'	☐	☐
Find a buddy or coach to work with on this	☐	☐
Keep a journal	☐	☐
Make self-care a priority	☐	☐
Say 'No' once more each day	☐	☐

Create a half hour of STOP time each week	☐	☐
Appreciate good service	☐	☐
Connect with people more often	☐	☐
Ask five people what your strengths are	☐	☐
Look to use your strengths more	☐	☐
Do more flow activities	☐	☐
Stop saying 'should', 'ought', 'can't', 'always', 'never'	☐	☐
Keep a gratitude journal	☐	☐
Stop trying to be consistent and be more spontaneous	☐	☐
Fix problems by giving them more time than they merit	☐	☐
Unpick areas of 'stuckness'	☐	☐
Take more considered risks	☐	☐
Sort out your doubts	☐	☐
Choose to be happy each day	☐	☐
Set small goals and make quick progress	☐	☐
Set out to have a great year	☐	☐
List 100 wants for your lifetime	☐	☐
List six things for the next day	☐	☐
Change how you handle your children	☐	☐
Ask for help	☐	☐

It's time to do a plan.

1. Pick the ideas that you have the most energy for –
   use the checklist above. Remember to modify them
   to suit your needs better if they do not fit at first.
2. Get a friend, a group of friends or a coach to help
   keep you focused. You can do this alone but progress
   will be a lot faster if you have company, someone
   walking alongside. You will also be paying the other

people a huge compliment if you tell them that you chose them because you wanted to do this with them. (If you would like some guidelines on how to form and run a group of people to do the work in this book then e-mail energygroup@coachingdirectors.com.)

3. Give them a chance to read this book and set up a time to talk through your impressions and preferences.

4. Pick a priority for you to work on, preferably the same one. Set a theme for the month, for example 'Clear the Clutter'.

5. Arrange a schedule for 'check-in' times, to compare progress and stay motivated. Make it a regular slot, something to look forward to, like lunch or a cup or drink of something after the gym.

6. Be ready to laugh.

7. Begin.

8. Take the time to notice the effect it has on you.

9. If you are willing, tell me how you get on. I will be inspired and tickled pink. Your results will boost my energy and could make my day. E-mail me at: energy@coachingdirectors.com.

We are all successful beyond measure. We are successful in the sense that we have created the circumstances in which we find ourselves. We may not actually like some of these circumstances, but that doesn't diminish our success in creating them. At some level, we wanted this, even if it *appears* not to serve us particularly well at the moment.

The invitation now is to fully accept that we are successful and therefore responsible, and then to ask ourselves:

would we like to be equally successful in creating some different circumstances? This is a powerful and energy-increasing way of looking at the world, our place within it and the opportunity before us right now.

Good luck, have fun and enjoy your energy!

RESOURCES

Sarah Ban Breathnach, *Simple Abundance*, Bantam (1995)

Steven Biddulph, *Raising Boys*, Thorsons (1997)

Paul Coelho, *Veronika Decides to Die*, HarperCollins (1998)

Stephen Covey, *First Things First*, Simon & Schuster (1994)

Stephen Covey, *The 7 Habits of Highly Effective People*, Simon & Schuster (1989)

Mihaly Csikszentmihalyi, *Flow – The Psychology of Optimal Experience*, Harper Perennial (1991)

Jinny Ditzler, *Your Best Year Yet*, Thorsons (1994)

Timothy Gallwey, *The Inner Game of Work*, Orion Business Books (2000)

Daniel Goleman, *Working with Emotional Intelligence*, Bloomsbury (1998)

Robert T. Kiyosaki, *Rich Dad, Poor Dad*, Warner (1997)

Nancy Kline, *Time to Think*, Ward Lock (1999)

Talane Miedaner, *Coach Yourself to Success*, Contemporary Books (2000)

Thomas Leonard, *The Portable Coach*, Scribner (1998)

Gregory McClellan Buchanan and Martin E. P. Seligman, eds, *Explanatory Style*, Lawrence Erlbaum Associates (1995)

Joseph O'Connor and John Seymour, *Introducing Neuro-Linguistic Programming*, Thorsons (1990)

Carl Rogers, *On Becoming A Person*, Constable (1974)

Bernie Siegel, *Prescriptions For Living*, Rider Books (1998)

John Whitmore, *Coaching for Performance*, Nicholas Brealey (1992)

Contacts

House of Colour, Esra Parr, Image Consultant
Tel: 020 8255 7280
E-mail: esra.parr@public-i.co.uk

The New Learning Centre
Tel: 020 7794 0321
E-mail: TNLC@dial.pipex.com
For courses on parenting skills

Organisations offering coach training
Coach U
www.coachu.com
In the UK contact Carol Golcher on 0800 0854 317.

CTI Co-Active Coaching
www.coaching-courses.com
Contact Estrella Associates on 01823 664 441.

The International Coach Federation
www.coachfederation.org
For additional organisations that train coaches.

ABOUT THE AUTHOR

Bill Ford is managing director of Coaching Directors, an organisation that specialises in coaching business people who want to be more effective *and* have a better balance between work and life. He sees his role as improving the bottom line by focusing on the people side of the business, and views increasing energy and resilience as crucial in creating desired results, both in work and in our personal lives.

Bill has worked in the US and in the UK in senior roles in marketing, advertising and market research. He has a degree in Psychology and is a certified practitioner in Neuro-Linguistic Programming.

Coaching Directors offers:

- executive coaching
- group and team coaching programmes
- workshops
- talks
- 360-degree feedback
- leadership development

For more general information on coaching and Coaching Directors, e-mail info@coachingdirectors.com.

For a free e-mail newsletter, please visit www.coaching directors.com.

For additional material not included in this book, visit www.coachingdirectors.com.